Healthy Lifestyle – Natural Tips to Live Healthy and Long

Ancient Health Tips and Techniques for a Healthy Life

Health Learning Series

Dueep Jyot Singh

Mendon Cottage Books

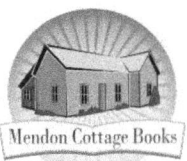

JD-Biz Publishing

All Rights Reserved.

No part of this publication may be reproduced in any form or by any means, including scanning, photocopying, or otherwise without prior written permission from JD-Biz Corp Copyright © 2015

All Images Licensed by Fotolia and 123RF.

Disclaimer

The information is this book is provided for informational purposes only. It is not intended to be used and medical advice or a substitute for proper medical treatment by a qualified health care provider. The information is believed to be accurate as presented based on research by the author.

The contents have not been evaluated by the U.S. Food and Drug Administration or any other Government or Health Organization and the contents in this book are not to be used to treat cure or prevent disease.

The author or publisher is not responsible for the use or safety of any diet, procedure or treatment mentioned in this book. The author or publisher is not responsible for errors or omissions that may exist.

Warning

The Book is for informational purposes only and before taking on any diet, treatment or medical procedure, it is recommended to consult with your primary health care provider.

Our books are available at

1. Amazon.com
2. Barnes and Noble
3. Itunes
4. Kobo
5. Smashwords
6. Google Play Books

Table of Contents

Introduction

Just go through any of the books, talking about the wisdom of the ages. You are going to find that longevity was the rule and not the exception. The allocated age of Three score and 10 given by nature to man was much more ages ago, because they had learned the rules of simple living in the most healthy manner possible.

Even though the 21st century may have its own accompanying health risks, including pollution, toxic waste, and other environmental problems, well calculated to make a human lifespan short, here are some ancient tips and techniques, which are still in use. All over the world, people are still following these common sense actions which can keep you healthy and increase your lifespan.

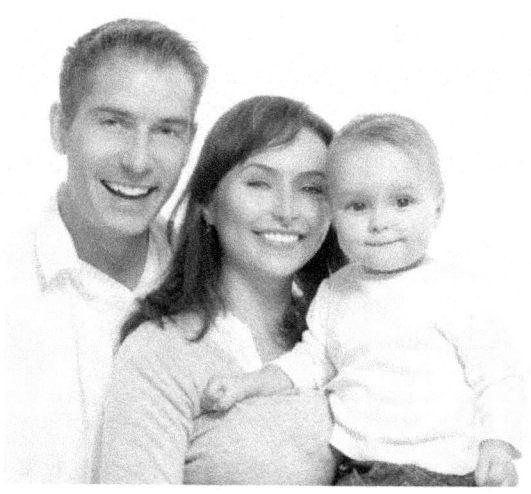

A healthy family is going to be a happy family

A great man once said "tell me what you eat and I will tell you what you are." So what we eat, and what we should not eat is going to have a very detrimental or very beneficial effect on our general state of health. What I ate as a child has kept me a comparatively healthy adult because fresh fruit and vegetables not only helped me grow in a healthy and normal fashion, but they also gave me a good strong immunity system. Along with that, I had plenty of fresh meat products, which provided me with healthy muscle building protein.

This was the diet which was eaten by the people of yore. And they ate their food in moderation. Often, they may not have had food to eat, because at that time, it was a clear case of survival of the fittest. But a missed meal once a day would have kept their systems healthy.

But today, thanks to the abundance of food in many parts of the world, we can be called gluttons. That is because we are so thankful to have good things to eat, that we eat, and we eat. And we eat. And that is going to have a bad effect on our general state of health, on a long-term basis.

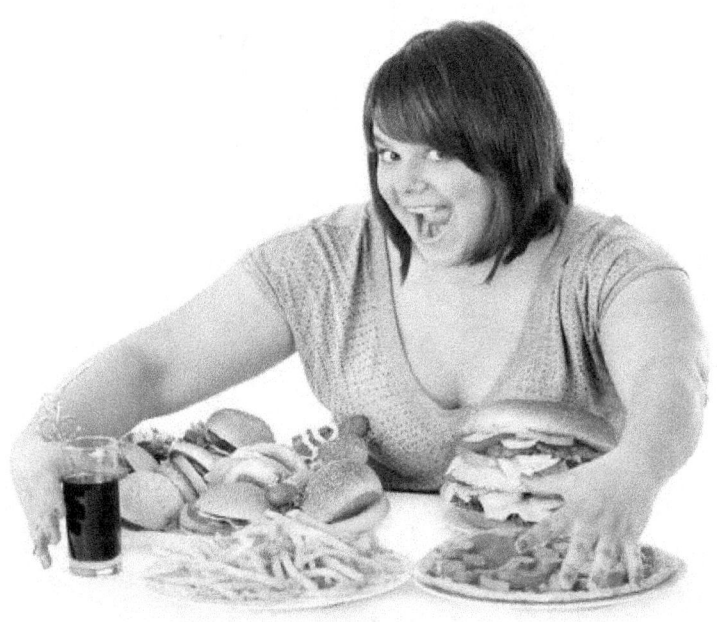

One of the subconscious reasons why we do not bother about our health is because we know that we have excellent medical facilities and doctors to take care of us in case we fall ill. Unfortunately, that is the lesson which is drilled into every child, the moment he begins to understand and assimilate the knowledge imparted to him by his parents. The parents are so used to running to the doctor for every single tiny ailment, that they do not allow nature to heal the child in its own special way. The doctor is going to give the child strong medicines, which is going to cure the child for a short-term, but may possibly have a future detrimental long-term effect on him.

But as we are used to quick results, we bother about the state of our health only when we find ourselves ailing or suffering from food related discomfort and problems. This has inconvenienced us; so it is time to go to the doctor.

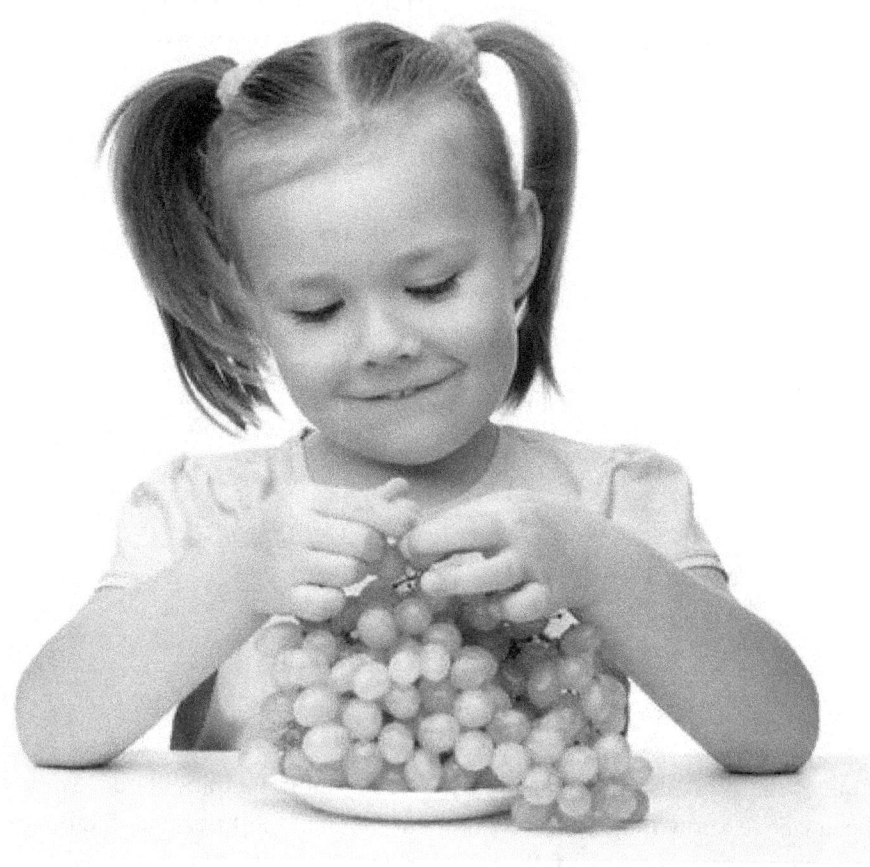

Healthy eating habits learned during childhood are going to keep this child healthy throughout her life.

Rules of Nutrition

Science has recognized the fact that the human body needs vitamins, proteins, carbohydrates, minerals, and other natural resources in order to keep functioning in a proper and healthy manner. I was astonished to see a number of my colleagues missing meals, and popping vitamin supplements, as a substitute.

Naturally I asked them why they were doing so, and why they were not getting their essential nutrients from healthy natural food items. They answered me that they were so used to popping pills, since childhood, that it had become a second habit. Also, who really had the time to eat real food in the shape of fresh fruit and vegetables and a home-cooked meal, when one was so busy busy busy at the office.

Unfortunately, this is not a rare occurrence in the world today. Most of us are doing exactly that. We are under the impression that supplements in the form of pills and other supplementary food products are going to keep us healthy, if we miss our meals.

That is so not true. It is also not right.

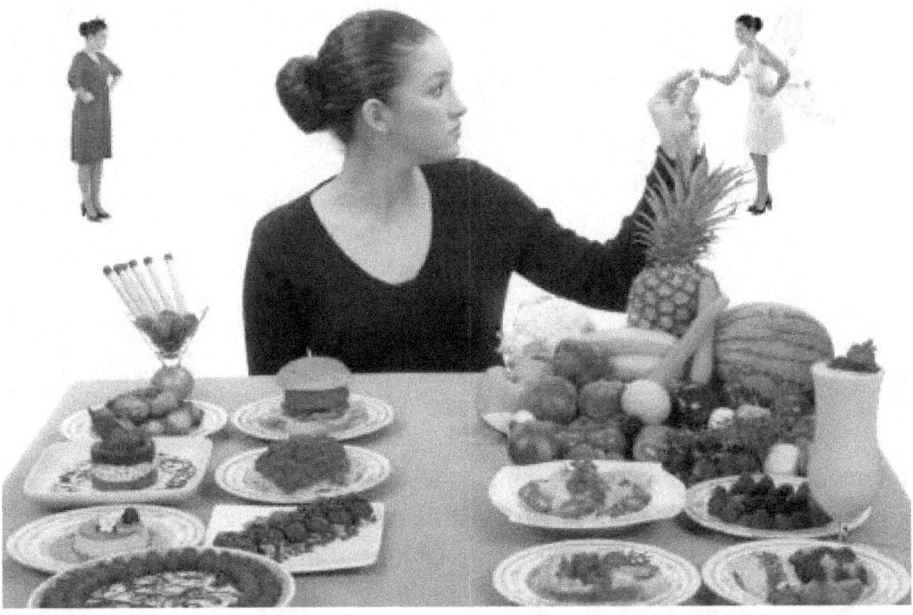

Remember that proper nutrition is the first safeguard to prevent you from illness. I asked a friend why she was not having regular meals and she made a face. Her landlady was a terrible cook. She did not know any place where she could get healthy meals. She could not cook herself, and besides, who had the time to do so? So she had begun skipping meals.

I never talked about the financial aspect of meals with her, but I know that in many cases, people skip meals, just because they cannot afford to eat. Now that is the sad thing, and I hope that is not the case with you.

This is definitely no excuse for you to neglect your health, just because you cannot find a good place, which can give you economical, tasty and nutritional meals.

Vegetarian Diet

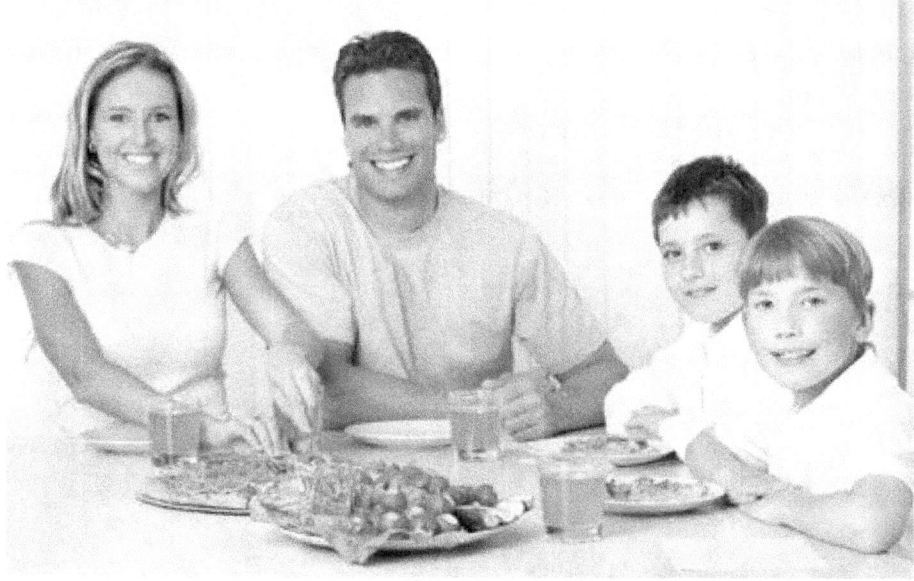

Let me give you an example of the benefits of a predominantly vegetarian diet.

In the late 50s, the Indian government selected my father for a USA government-sponsored steel training and educational program held in the CASE Inst. of technology, Cleveland, Ohio, and in other places all over the country and in Canada. Father was a prey to ill health, chronic cough and cold since childhood, but he went off adventuring to the USA with gusto. He had been born under A Wandering Star, always ready for new experiences.

During his stay in the USA and Canada, he had to spend a few months in New York. The Government "stipend"was enough to survive in Cleveland, but it was definitely not enough for New York. With the aim of completing his training successfully, he did not complain about the limited budget. And he liked to eat, especially when his health started improving the moment he reached the USA and he found himself changing his diet out of necessity!

That meant he needed to sacrifice the "taste" part of his food while switching over to a more balanced nutritional and least expensive food items.

So whenever he was sent to train in a new city, the first thing he did was check out the Chinese restaurants there on the roadside. They were just coming into prominence, as roadside stalls, and for about USD.50, he had a huge meal prepared right in front of him. That was his lunch. For breakfast, he had bread, butter and toast, bacon and eggs. Eggs and white meat were an essential part of his diet. Apart from that, he had his fill of Californian oranges, and other delicious citrus fruit, or any other locally available fruit and vegetables, whenever he could.

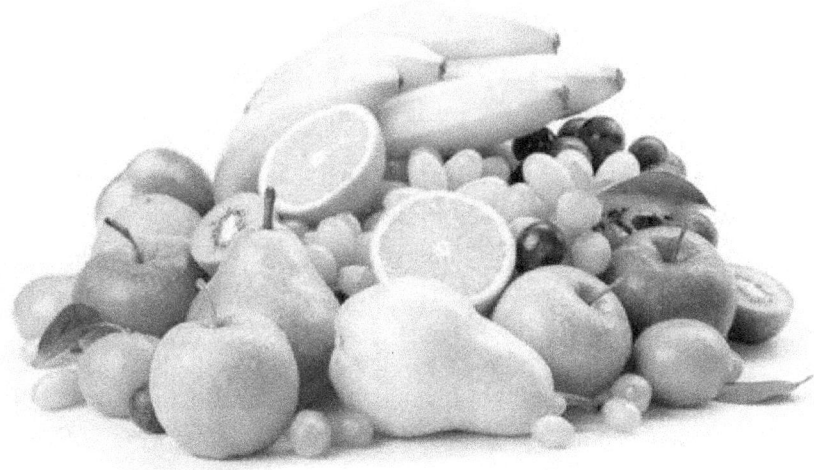

He also had jumbo sandwiches at automats, which were filled with nutritional fillings like lettuce, butter, cheese, chicken, and occasionally ham, and mayonnaise. Delicatessens also provided him with many inexpensive meals.

Meat was considered necessary only to balance the nourishing constituents of the food. Chicken was comparatively inexpensive when compared to Pork, lamb and beef. So he had chicken whenever he could.

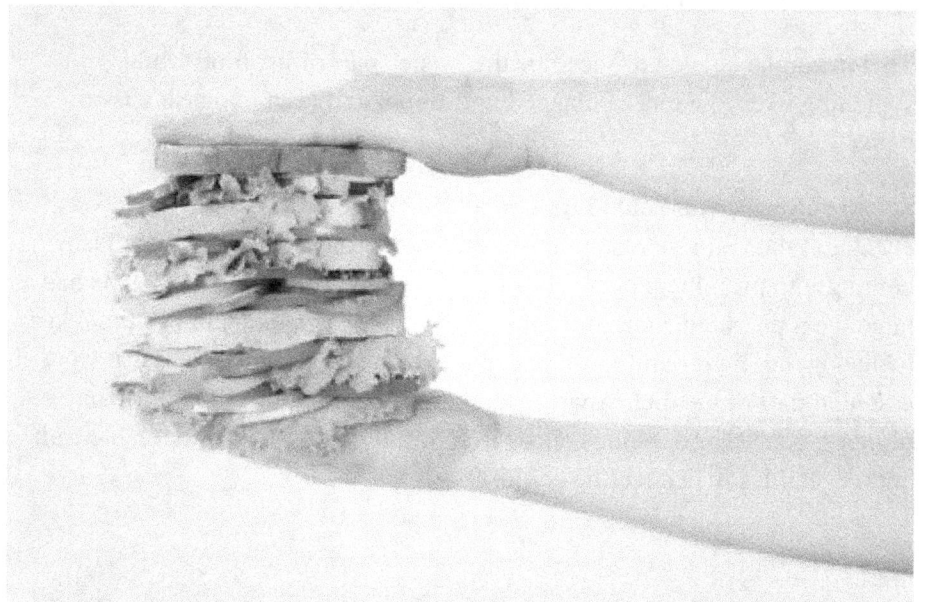

A jumbo chicken sandwich with all the four food groups, along with lots of greens can help ward off the hunger pangs.

During the mandatory and prescribed medical examination necessary during the course of the training, the doctor talked to my father after an x-ray examination. He told him that his "chest was okay." And then he asked him how he had got rid of pleurisy, because the doctor had seen the scars on father's lungs!

Believe it or not, this healthy diet for one whole year of fruit and vegetables, meat and cereal, and other natural food items without any preservatives, had cured him completely of incipient pleurisy which by the way, he did not know he had! These had been completely healed. It was at that time that he understood that his cough and cold was due to this serious ailment and his frequency of bouts had almost finished during his stay there.

By the time he came back to India, his persistent and very troublesome cough and cold were things of the past, never to return again, even though since then, he spent his life in high-altitude areas where harsh winter weather and rain throughout the year was expected and accepted with relish.

He attributes this cure to his diet – mainly vegetarian with lots of vegetables and fruit. The main aim was nutrition and not lots of taste enhancing preservatives and additives.

Also, he never took any vitamins, supplements, medicines, drugs, and any other prescriptions recommended to him by doctors, all the time he was there.

Our ancestors lived in this manner. They did not go asking for sulfa drugs and other chemical-based drugs for a small sniffle. They let nature take her time and cure them.

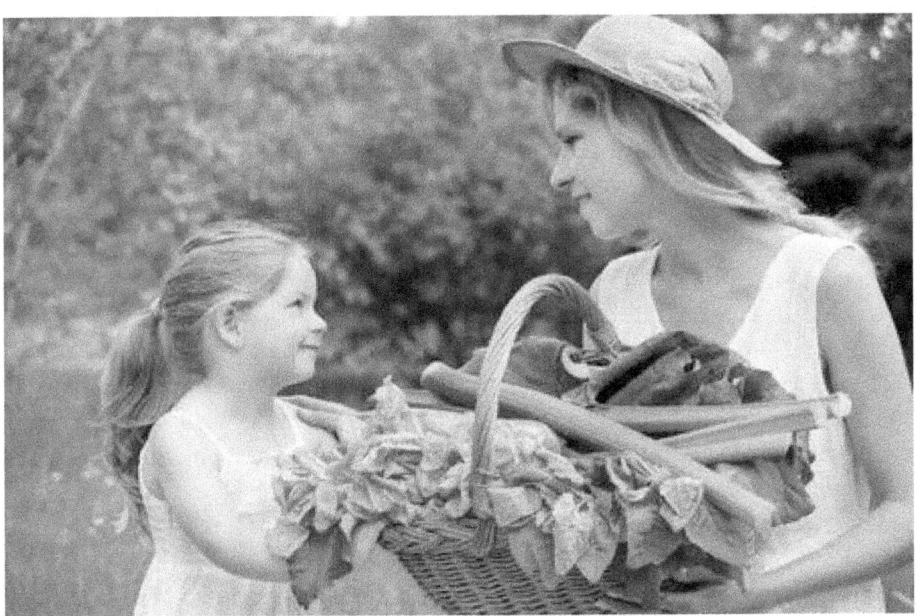

Our ancestors appreciated the value of green vegetables and leafy plants. This is one of the sensible ideas passed down to us, which, thankfully, we have not discarded as being too old school.

This also shows that man who is supposed to have acquired his taste for non- vegetarian foods through his simian evolutionary genes should remember that monkeys are not normally non-vegetarian. They do eat meat when they can get it, but they subsist more on roots, fruit and vegetables. That is why they are genetically healthy and constitutionally sturdy. They are also physically more active and energetic when compared to human beings.

And this is the diet which has kept father so healthy, even though he is 84 now and by the grace of that diet – and possibly his ancestral genes –, he is still going strong and still goes somersaulting in the swimming pool. [1]

And I do not have to fear that in the winter, he is going to come down with cough, cold, chest pain, or any such problems, ever. Naturally, we are still occasionally non vegetarian, especially in the winter, but that is to keep the protein level high. His diet was very simple in the USA. It still is.

---

[1] 10 years ago he volunteered to teach the children and teenagers of the area how to swim, because swimming is something their parents had not learned. I am preparing a video to be uploaded on YouTube, with him diving, floating, somersaulting, and swimming underwater, while training children and youngsters, out of which one teenager has already reached the state levels swimming team! So that is the life lived Emperor size, according to father.

The purpose of the video is just to show how effective a healthy diet is for people, even in their 80s, and how that diet can be followed by anyone, anywhere in the world.

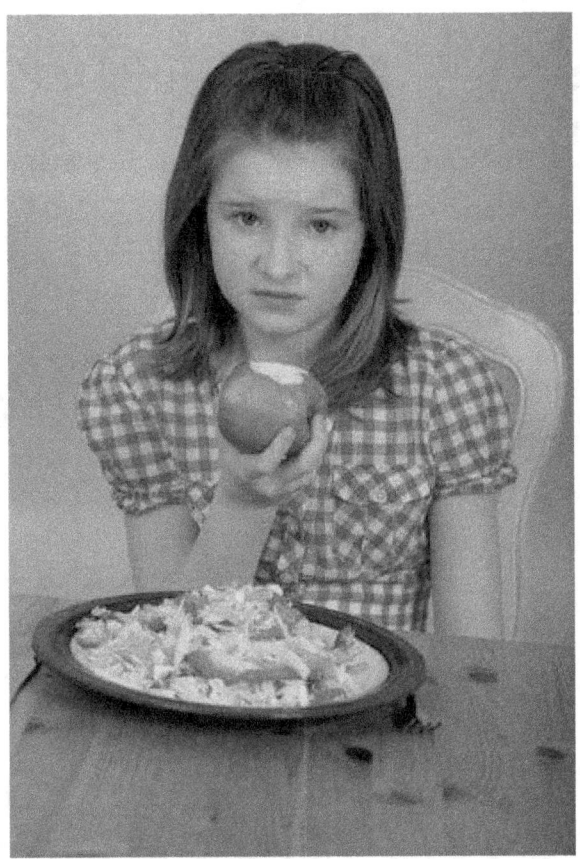

Many children just hate eating fruit and vegetables, because their parents force them to do so, saying "you have to eat it, because it is good for you." Are you doing this to your child?

Also, even though father is not a teetotaler, he avoided drinking alcoholic products throughout his life as far as he could. Tea, coffee, and milk, along with water, provide him with necessary fluids.

So what had happened to boost up his immunity system in such a manner? A steady, regular diet of healthy nutritional food. A healthy lifestyle with plenty of exercise – walking from one place to the other in the cities of the 30 countries he visited, since then, to save transport money – and absolutely no recourse to doctors or prescription drugs.

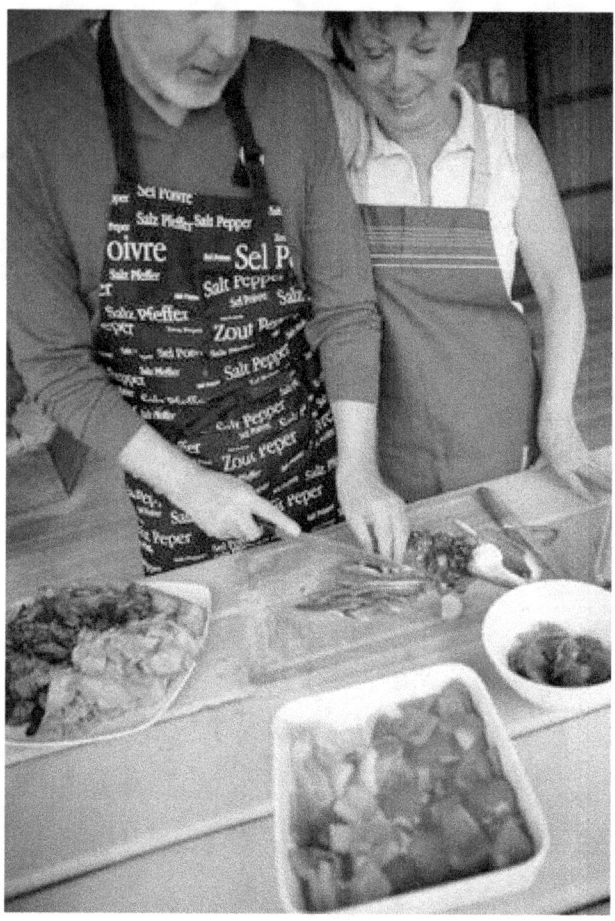

Also, he never eats any food item with chemical taste makers like monosodium glutamate – aji-no-moto – added to them. You must be aware that some of the international popular food brands have a cautionary warning that children below is certain age group should not be given this food because of the monosodium glutamate. That should make you realize the truth behind preservation and also proves the point of a beneficial nutritional diet to give you a long-term healthy Constitution.

So Why Do We Fall Sick?

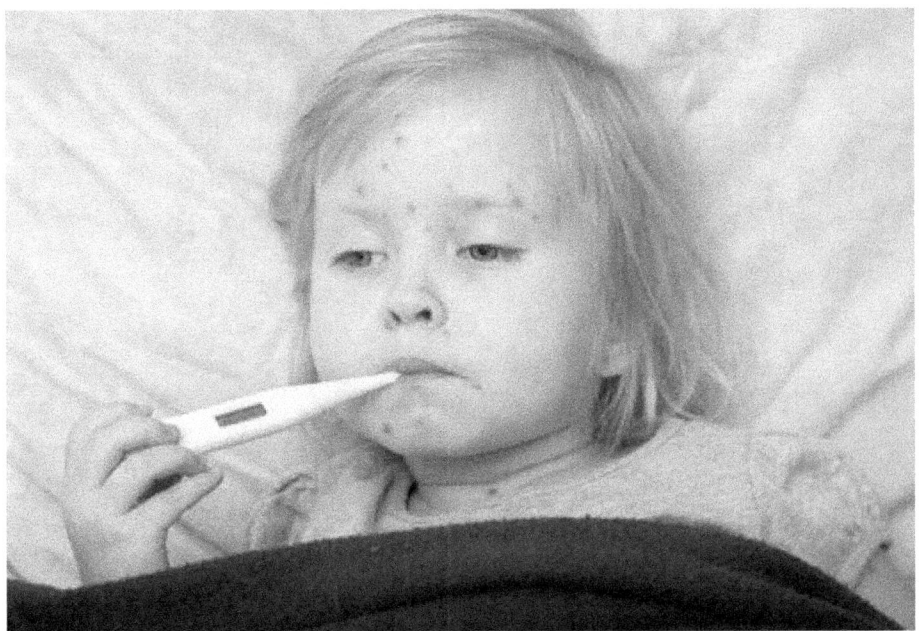

To get a totally nutritionally balanced diet, we need necessary nutrients in our daily diet, which are going to keep our system working properly. These include carbohydrates, vitamins, proteins, fats, minerals, and other essential nutrients which we get from our food. Any sort of deficiency in any of these items is going to cause malnutrition. They are also going to make us more prone and vulnerable to diseases.

In olden times a person who was sick was healed by his cooks, instead of his doctors. In ancient Korean and Japanese history, families who could afford experienced and much in demand cooks always had them to keep the whole family healthy. These cooks were trained in the art of healing through food. They knew the Constitution and system of each family member. They knew which foods suited him best. They also knew that if some family member was suffering from some particular ailment, it was because he was suffering from some sort of deficiency in his food.

A good digestive system kept all these people healthy and long-lived. Consider food to be a natural medicine, which is going to you and keep you healthy.

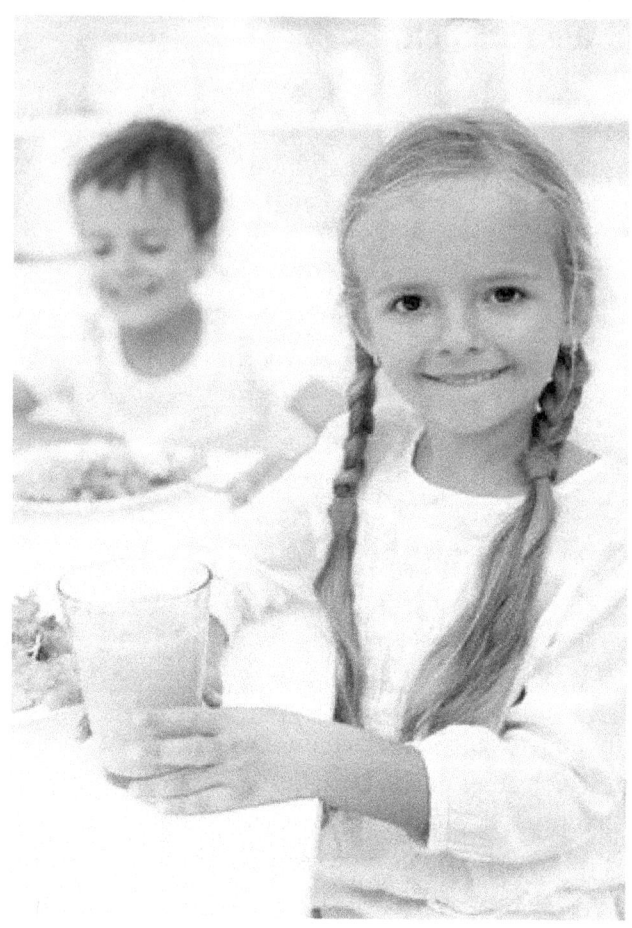

Changing your lifestyle and changing your diet is something which you are not going to do overnight. It took you six months to get that extra flabby tire on your tummy. That was because you change your diet pattern and decided that exercise was a bore. Your body took six months to get this message and the spare tire showed up accordingly.

The ancients took a long time over their meals. These were leisurely activities, and every morsel was chewed properly and carefully. If the food is natural, and organic, it is going to assimilate even better in your system.

Deficiency of vitamin C in food is something which causes most of our ailments. In the 14th, 15th and 16th century sailors in many parts of Europe suffered a lot from scurvy. That is because their food during long voyages was boiled meat and hardtack biscuits. So the moment they reached sunny shores, they found the state of their health improving, because they were eating those native exotic fruit in large quantities.

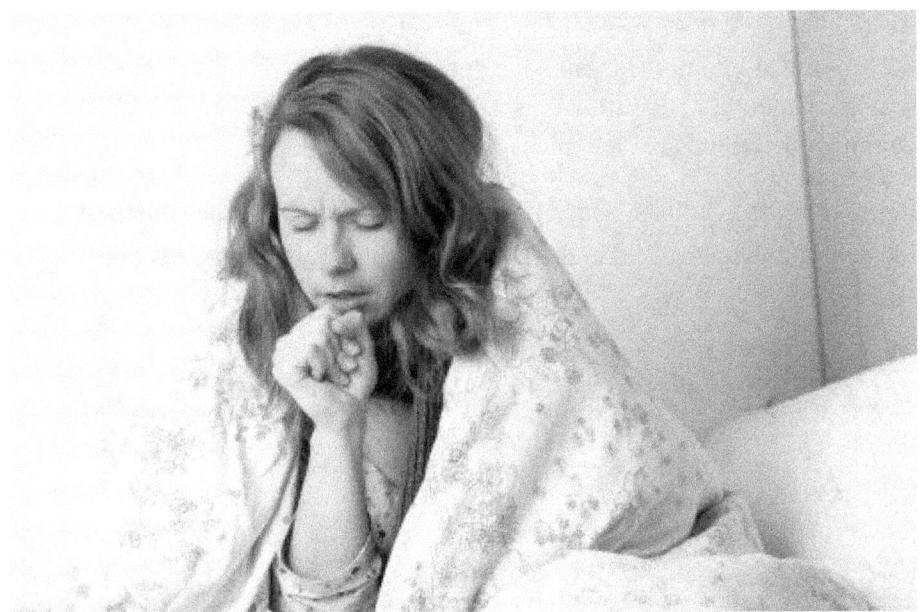

Persistent coughs and colds in the winter means you are suffering from low vitamin C deficiency.

But Portuguese sailors did not suffer from such health problems, even during long sea voyages. That is because they put large chunks of meat and pork and lots of garlic in wooden casks, and barrels. They would then fill these up with vinegar. The vinegar prevented the food from spoiling, and the garlic provided all the sailors with necessary minerals and nutrients to keep them healthy.

So when other European navies found their sailors falling sick due to bad nutrition, and also malnutrition because they had run out of food, the Portuguese were successful in making colonies all over the world, thanks to meat preserved naturally, vinegar and garlic.

The lack of vitamin C showed up in other sailors in a pale complexion, fatigue and lethargy, pain in the muscles, swollen and bleeding gums and dental problems like pyorreah and falling teeth. Also, their wounds did not heal properly and naturally, and their bones were brittle and fragile. Their immunity system grew weaker and the body fell prey to diseases. They also suffered from cold, cough, pneumonia and other chest infections very often.

Just imagine all these problems due to the lack of one small vitamin. The best source of vitamin C is cabbage, lettuce, citrus fruits like lemons, oranges, limes, etc., cauliflower, small carrots, onions, tomatoes, radishes, coriander, beetroot, spinach, pineapples and Guavas.

Here is one ancient herb which has been considered to be the source of longevity, down the ages, in the East. It is called **The Gooseberry** – Amla-.

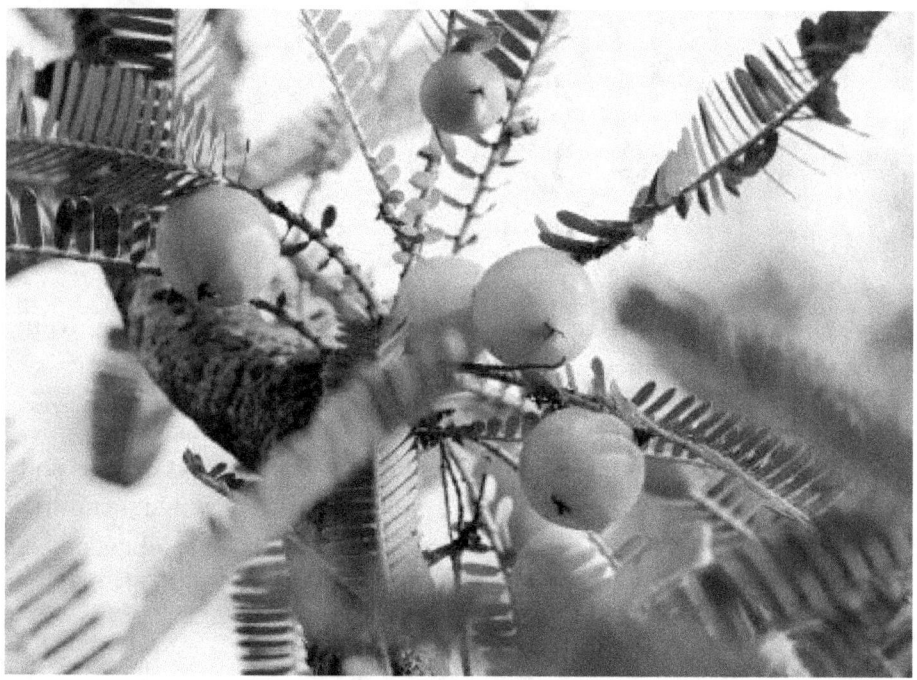

Not only is it considered to be an excellent health food, but it is instrumental in keeping the ladies of the East beautiful because of its wonderful skin toning and hair tonic qualities.

It can either be eaten raw, in dried and powdered form, or you can cook it. I remember eating this fruit in large quantities as a kid, even though the sour taste was one acquired. Thanks to this, my teeth are still healthy and I have never had to visit a dentist.

I am referring to perpetually hungry kids eating guavas and gooseberries, whenever and wherever they could get them. We did not bother much about the medicinal value at that time. But for millenniums, this particular fruit has been used to improve your appetite, and your immunity system, give you a healthy sleep, help in your powers of concentration and get rid of headaches and also darkens your hair naturally. It also gives your hair a natural shiny luster.

So if you have access to real gooseberry powder – just dry it, grind it and filter it in a fine cloth – take 1 teaspoon with one teaspoonful of honey every morning for about four months. Four months is more than enough to you of many problems, even though you are going to see visible results in a month or so.

Why did I say four months, you may ask? These ancient remedies cured diseases from the roots. It took a while, but the results were long lasting and permanent. So many of us would be tempted to stop eating the Gooseberry honey mixture, after one month, because hey, our hair has already stopped falling, and it has started growing dark from the roots. Also, our skin looks so young and youthful. And so on.

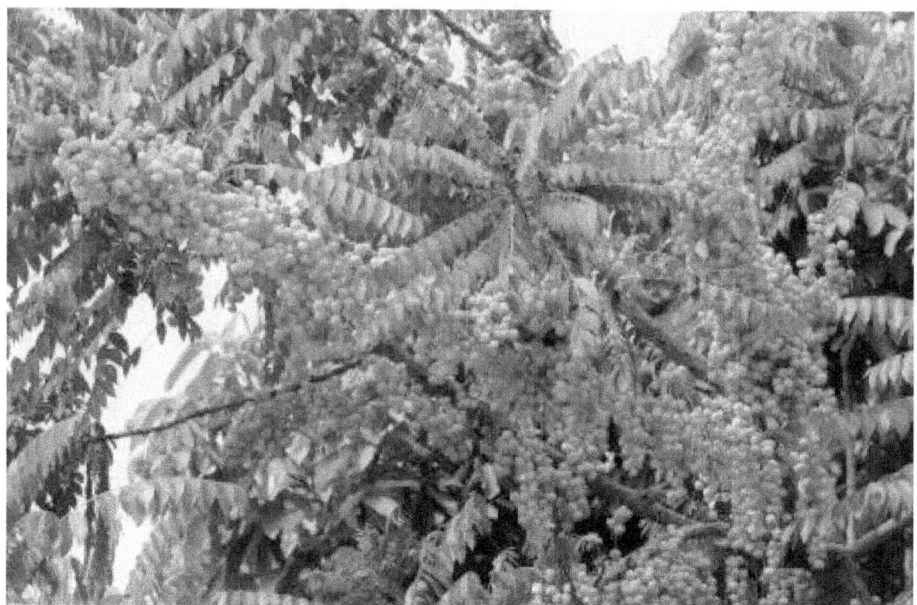

But the four months treatment is to tone up your system from the roots. It just takes one minute, so instead of popping a vitamin pill, pop a spoonful of gooseberry powder mixed with a spoonful of honey. And wait for the results.

But if you are too busy to do that, here is another ancient recipe to keep you healthy and to give you the best natural vitamin C supplement – gooseberry.

Make a number of pills with this powder, mixing it with water and honey. Brown organic sugar , also known as jaggery, or Panela in Mexico and South America can also be used when you do not have honey around, and drying the pills in the shade. Six pills three times a day and hey presto, you are going to see a distinct improvement in your health. Within two months, you are going to find yourself more energetic and more vital and healthier.

Vitamin A is also an important nutrient which you need to have in your diet. Lack of vitamin A means weaker eyesight. You may also suffer from night blindness, your eyes feel dry and itchy. You may also find small pin head sized growths on your skin. Your teeth and gums are going to be affected. The moment you find yourself suffering from a vitamin A deficiency, start adding cabbage, coriander, mint, green leaves of radishes, fenugreek, spinach, carrot, and papayas to your diet.

All the vegetables given above can be eaten raw. You can also use them as salads or blended in vegetable cocktails. You can also drink their juices. Try the addition of these vegetables to your diet, and it is a proven fact that within three months, you are going to see a distinct cure of these particular health problems.

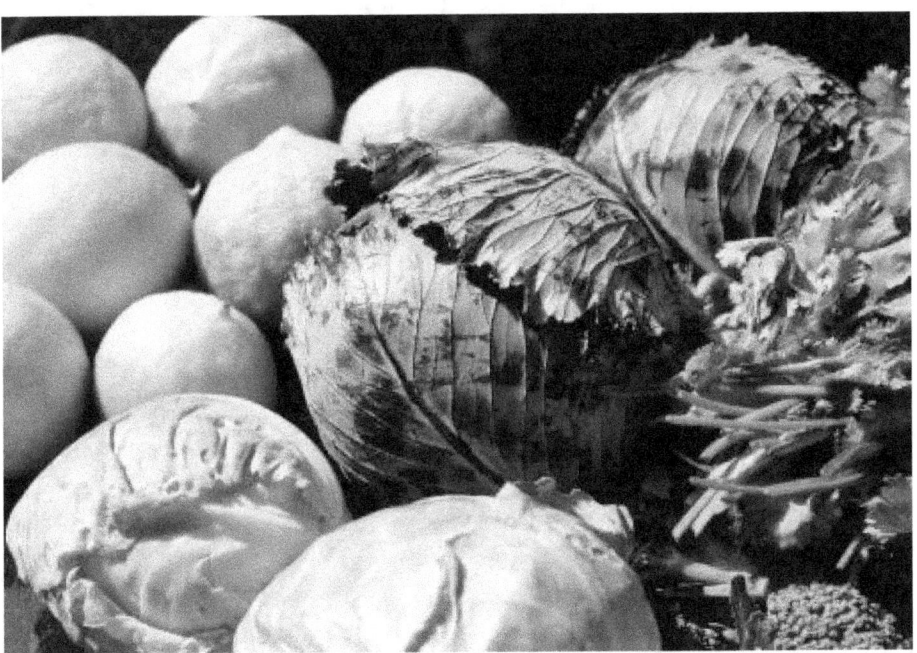

How to Use Fruit and Vegetables Effectively

For people suffering from digestive problems, start drinking the juice of fruit and vegetables diluted in water. This natural juice therapy is going to take a little while before it starts to take effect. That is because your body is coming back to its natural state of good health. Slowly and steadily, you are going to find yourself getting cured of ailments, thanks to this therapy.

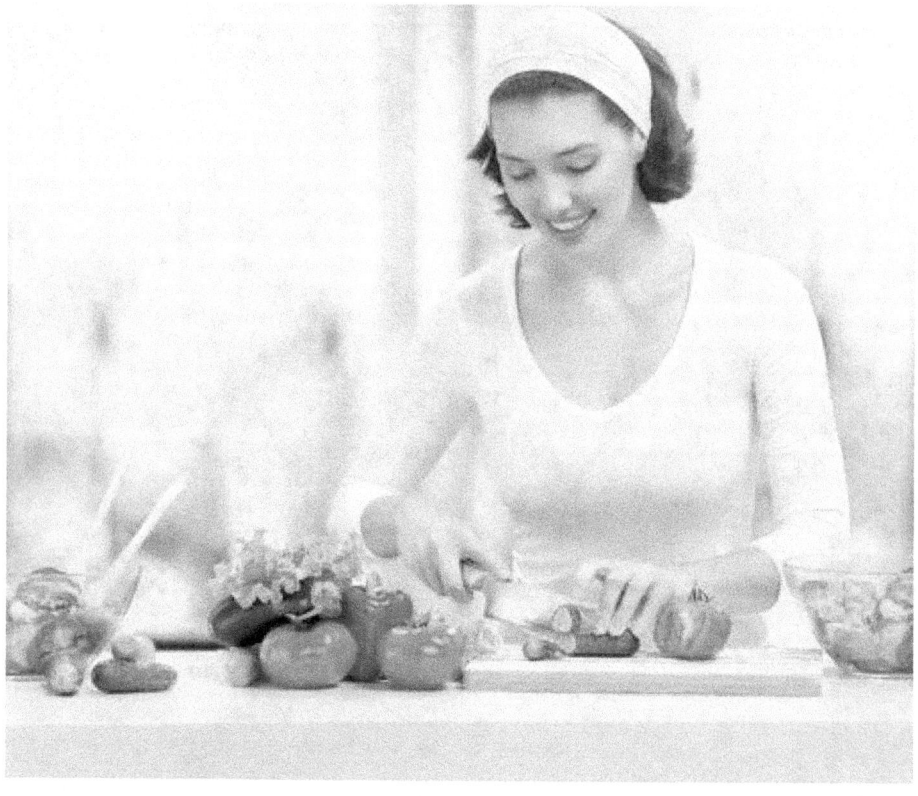

I remember meeting a cousin after a long time at a wedding. She was getting married in the next three months. Her mother had already enrolled her in a naturopathic farm in the city, where she was put on a fruit and vegetable diet. Her skin glowed, but she said that she had been drinking fruit and vegetable juice for the past 20 days, and it was such a blessing to manage to use the excuse of another relative's wedding to escape from the juice diet.

At least now she could eat everything she wanted to her heart's delight. And alas, she would be going back to durance vile, the next day, to that naturopathy retreat. But when I told her that she looked absolutely beautiful, she cheered up and began to look forward to that fruit and vegetable diet again.

In ancient times, this tradition was part of the East, before a wedding. The bride would be fed a special diet made up of vegetables and fruit. She would not be given "hot" spices, meat, eggs, and herbs like garlic and onions.

Drink the juice in the morning and in the afternoon. You can take 16 ounces of juice every day in one sitting. Eat the vegetables and fruit according to their seasonal appearance during the year and do not eat unseasonable vegetables like mangoes and pineapples in the winter exported from abroad at high costs.

Start reducing the intake of sugar. The body is quite capable of manufacturing its own requirement of sugar from the food we eat, all on its own. Some of us say that we have a sweet tooth and that is our excuse to eat lots of sugary items. In fact, we are overdosing ourselves on sugar. This artificially produced and defined sugar is definitely harmful.

If you really want to sweeten something, use honey. Do not tip in a full teaspoonful into your drink, all at once. Try half a teaspoonful at first. You may find yourself getting accustomed to half a teaspoonful and the tasty drink thus ensuing.

Food Peelings

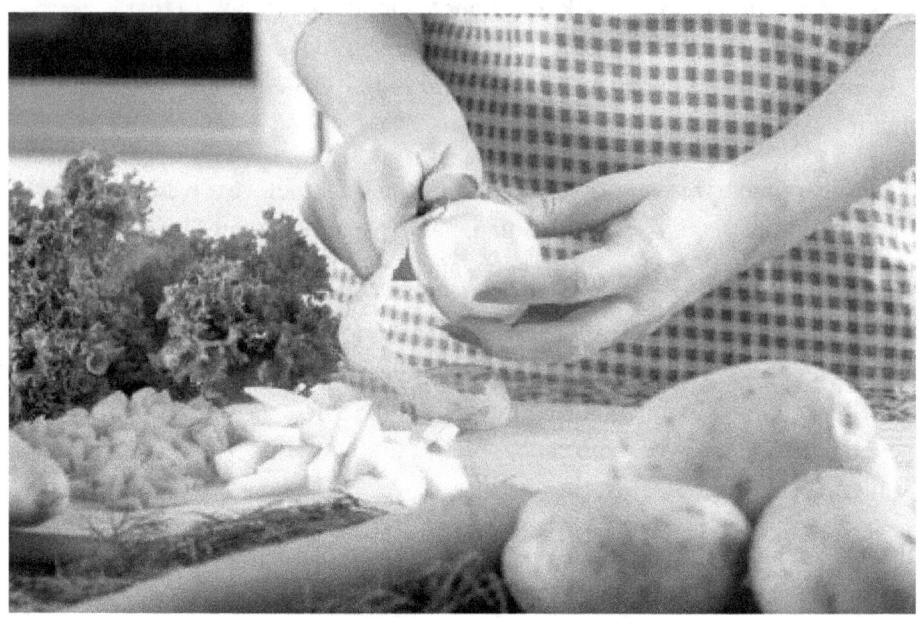

Peeling the potato means losing all those nutrients

If the outer peel or skin is not very hard, you can eat the fruit or the vegetable along with the skin. Hey, you say, you mean you can eat oranges and lemons, along with the skin?

Of course, if there have been grown organically and you know that they are not inundated with toxic pesticides. Just remember to wash them properly. I have seen commuters on buses in London, busily munching away oranges from brown paper bags, and though I was surprised because that was the first time I had seen somebody eating something with the skin on, I did not dare to tell the lady that she had not washed the orange.

I would be told in no uncertain terms to MYOBB or even to Fuh Cough, depending on her mood, her command over the language, and her upbringing.

Did you know that potato peelings have a major part of the nutrients in them? So have cucumber peelings and Apple peelings. But the first thing we do is go on eBay and buy a really nice fruit and vegetable peeler, for

USD.25, Buy Now, free international shipping. Who could resist a bargain, such as that? And once it is in our hands, we use it on the surface of every available vegetable and fruit being washed and scrubbed and peeled under the tap.

What a waste of natural nutrients. No wonder potatoes baked in their skins are a well-known and popular dish. Remember that if you feel any sort of problem on eating any fruit and vegetable, stop eating it right now. There may be a chance that that particular food item does not suit your bio – physiological system and constitution.

Diseases and Diet Control

There are some rules which have been followed since ancient times, which have helped people keep up a healthy lifestyle. These are easy to utilize tips which you can start doing or following immediately.

Drink three mouthfuls of water, before you eat something. This is going to lubricate your food passage, and get your digestive system ready for the well chewed material which is going to be digested in the stomach and the intestines.

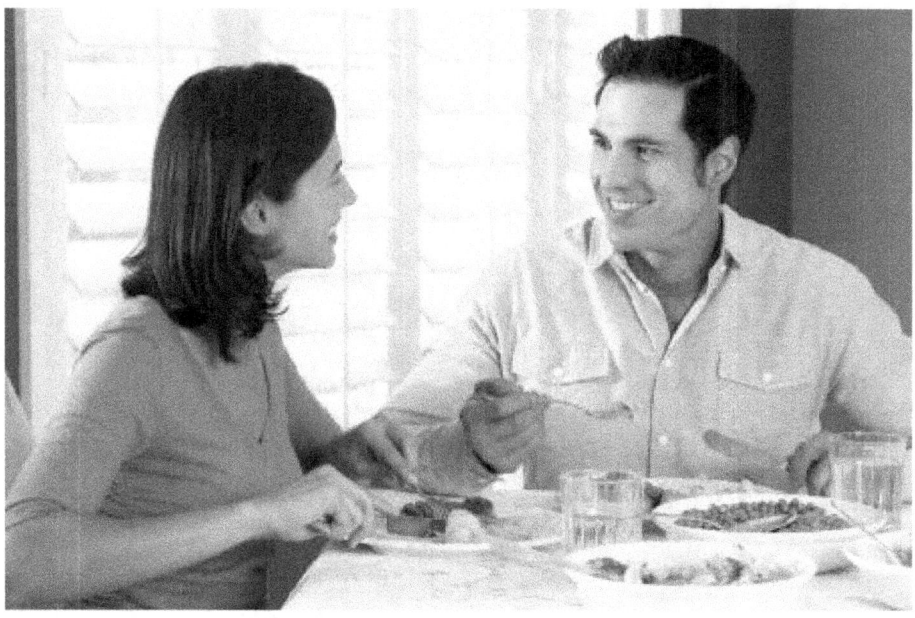

Believe it or not, most of the modern medicines do not cure sicknesses. They just make the ailments go away temporarily, and the symptoms are not visible. The root of the sickness is still there somewhere, just waiting for an opportunity to pounce, especially if you are not healthy.

Along with that, these modern medicines have such long-lasting side effects that you need to take more medicine in order to get rid of the side effects. The new medicines are going to have even more side effects, and then you are going to take more medicines to cure the side effects of the side effects of the original disease. This is going to go on ad infinitum.

However, diseases can be controlled and kept in check with a strict dietary regimen. If you have an unhealthy lifestyle, it is going to show up in your health.

Let me tell you one secret why people living thousands of years ago were so healthy compared to us? That is because they did their food raw as far as possible. This meant minimum cooking. And it also meant more of raw fruit and vegetables, nuts, grains and other easily digestible food.

This rule shows that they do not eat too much meat, because that needed to be cooked. But as man began to be civilized, he started adding pulses and beans to his diet, which needed to be cooked to be digested. And so the state of his natural health started deteriorating and in a couple of millenniums, he started suffering from digestion related diseases.

Reducing Your Weight

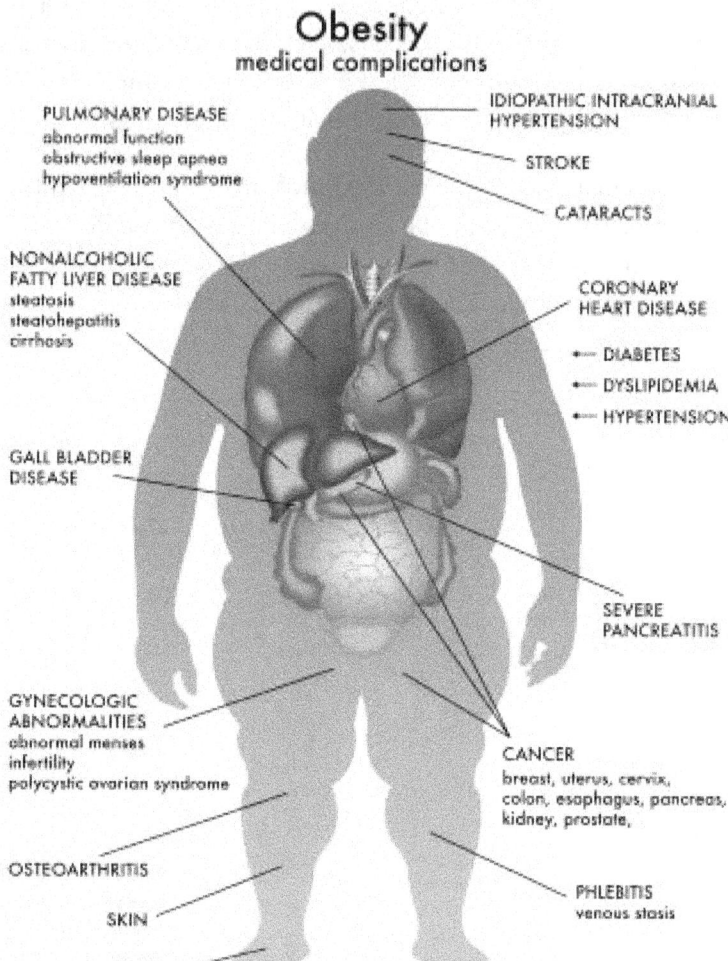

One knows for a fact that obesity is related to a number of diseases. These include heart attacks, high blood pressure, liver problems, diabetes, potential stroke, gout and lethargy.

It is quite difficult to reduce weight, once you put it on, so that is why prevention is better than cure. The stop line for men is 155 pounds and 130 pounds for women. This is a general estimate, and it is going to vary, increasing or lessening, depending on your height. The moment you find yourself going over that line, it is time to put a stop to your eating binges

If you have a sedentary lifestyle, you are going to need only 1500 – 2000 cal in your diet. Anything above this is going to add to the fat content in your body. 3000 – 4000 cal and more is what are needed by people who have an active lifestyle. That is so that they can get enough of energy to keep functioning in a healthy, natural way.

However, even though most of us follow a sedentary lifestyle, our calorie intake is that of people following active lifestyles. That is because the food is in front of us and we insist on emptying out our overloaded plates because who knows, we might feel hungry even after we have eaten, and we do not like that sensation!

These are the foodstuffs which contribute to fat – red meat, butter and other high-fat containing dairy products, rice, fried stuff, sweet dishes, sugar, grapes, and even bananas in excess.

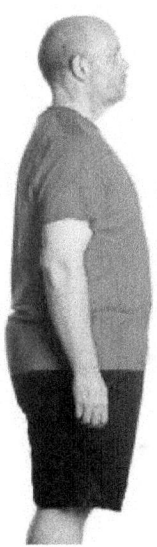 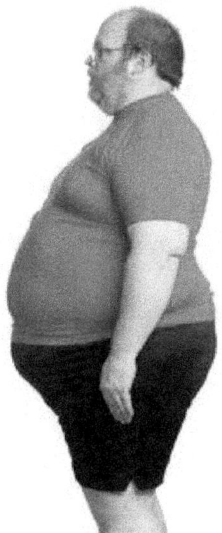

Also, the ancients say that if you sleep in the afternoons, keep eating throughout the day, and do not move about enough, you are going to get fat.

Aha, is that why the lovely señoritas of Mediterranean countries are so well-rounded – is the siesta to blame?

I could not care less, I cannot do without my restoring siesta!

So here is the reducing weight regime.

Do not overload your plate. You can always go back for second helpings. You may not want to do that, surprisingly enough, once you have finished everything on your plate. Well, this is mental autosuggestion with your stomach telling your brain that you have done with the eating process!

Drink water after an hour of eating. Also, if you have to take a bath, have a bath an hour after you have taken a meal, and with cold water.

Do a little bit of fasting.

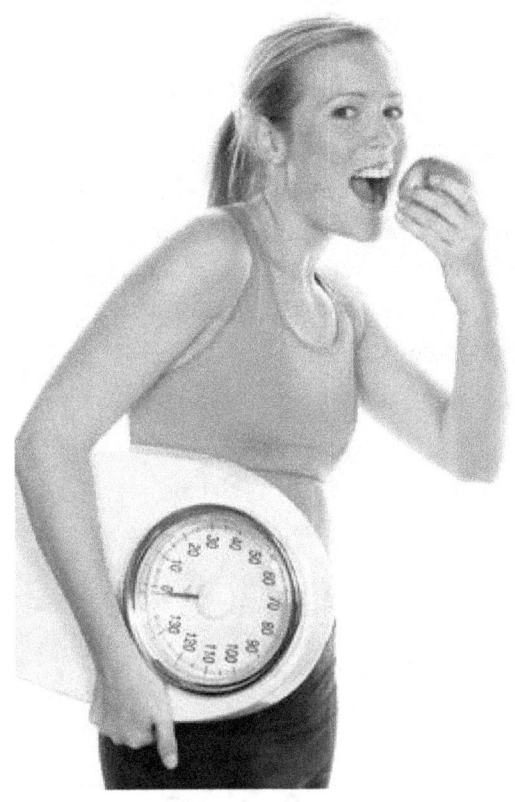

No meals, or just a fruit diet can help keep the weight down.

Now what is fasting? That is missing a meal on purpose, about once a week in order to get your system toned up again. But if you are in the habit of missing meals regularly, because you are too busy to eat, do not fast. That is because all those missed meals already come under the category of fasting and they are going to soon bring you to the stage of possible starvation.

Fasting is done as a religious practice in many parts of the world. Well, this is a good way to achieve mental, emotional, spiritual and physical well-being, all at the same time.

Also, remember to leave the table, before you consider yourself totally satiated. You need to be just a little bit hungry before you stop eating. I found that a sedentary lifestyle had made me put on weight. So I decided to read the day's choice of book when eating. And I did not get to know that I had finished up my smaller portions of lunch and dinner. When the plate was empty, all right, I had finished eating.

Surprisingly enough, I never felt as if I was feeling hungry even after I had finished my meal.

Try a total fruit diet for a couple of weeks. This can only be done if you have access to lots of fruit. During that time, you are going to drink fruit juice and you are not going to eat cereals, milk products, rice, sugar and sweet stuff. Look at the difference after 10 days of juice, fruits and vegetables eaten raw or in salads.

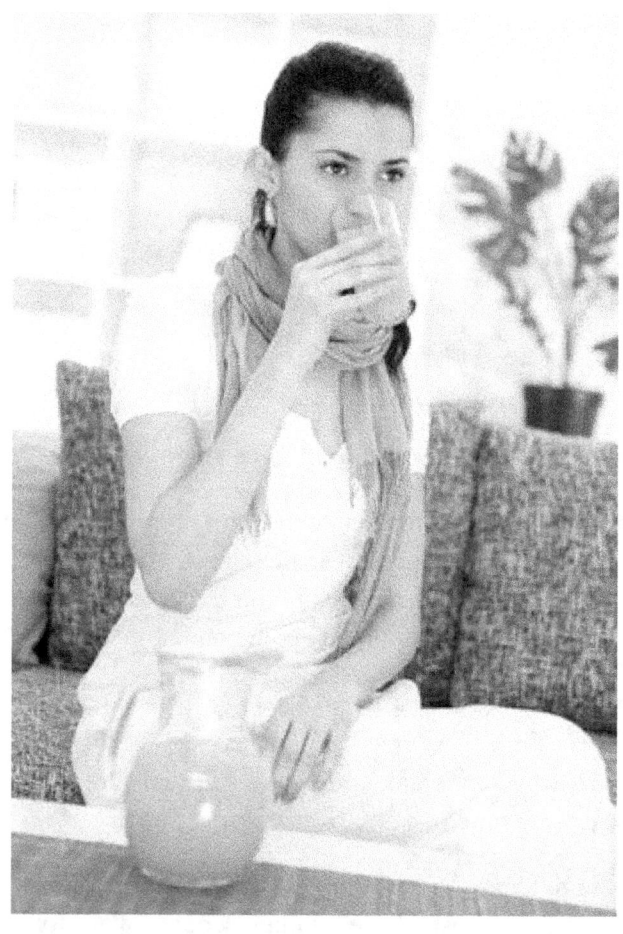

Regular exercise and massage also helps break down the fat cells in the body. That is because the muscular tissues get into action. They need more oxygen because you are subjecting them to an unusual and unused – to activity. So they need more energy. They are going to get that energy from the fat cells.

So try a regular exercise routine. Walking at a leisurely pace does not work. But a half jog half trot is more beneficial. Swimming, dancing, and other physical activities can help you lose weight.

Dancing is not an exercise! It is pure fun even though the calisthenics, stretch, bend, and other dancing gestures you are going through remind you of the physical training exercises you did at School and University! They were so boring, 1234, and your instructor blowing the whistle and yelling at you.

On the other hand, a dance instructor going 1234 does not seem to have that same monotonous and "gleeep" effect on your mind and showing in your face. That is the reason why so many of us enjoy dancing so much. That is because our minds know that dancing is a fun activity, and not a boring exercise!

Relaxation is the best way to reduce weight. You are de-stressing yourself. Your circulation tones itself up. The toxic wastes in your body get eliminated as you take deep breaths and let your muscles fall loose.

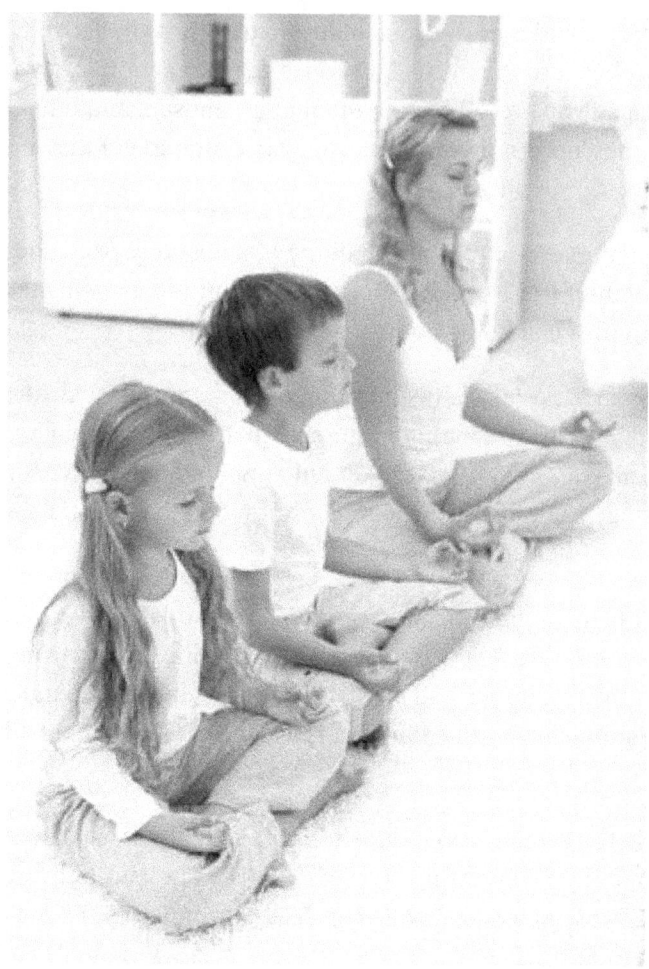

Also, here is another tip. Add the calcium intake in your body. Researchers say that calcium produces some sort of hormone which is good for your metabolism. A good metabolism is going to burn calories. This means that the fatty cells are going to reduce themselves, slowly and steadily.

So try it out, start eating more calcium rich foods in your diet from today itself.

This URL is going to tell you more about calcium rich foods.

http://www.webmd.com/food-recipes/10-calcium-rich-foods

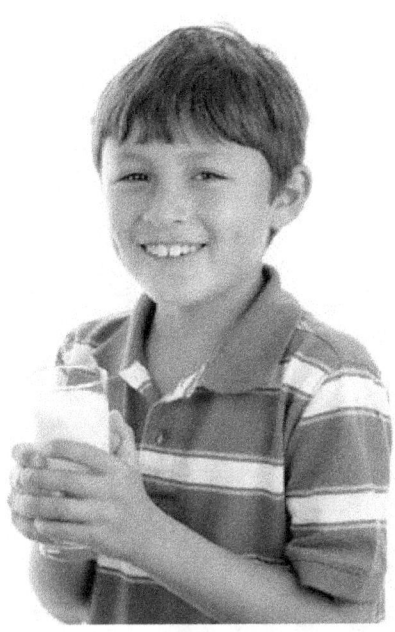

Cheese and dairy products are rich in calcium. So have as much of cheese as long as it is not processed, as you can. Milk is necessary for growing children

If you really do not have the time to go outside and do some exercise in the fresh air, at least spend 15 minutes a day doing some sort of vigorous activity, which helps burn off the calories. I enjoy reading novels, when the hero is so angry about something that he goes to the gym, and works out until he is all sweaty. This is a good way for him to cool off, because by the time he has exhausted himself, he is also thought things out.

So getting sweaty in the gym does not mean subjecting your body to trauma or getting your muscles so sore that waking up next day is sheer purgatory.

Exercise routines should always be done slowly and steadily. Anything that causes your body pain has to be stopped immediately. It is said that Bruce Lee did about 1000 push-ups every day. Now that is obsessiveness. That is also subjecting the body to too much exercise. At one time I used to walk anywhere between five – 15 km, just listening to music, in the park. That managed to burn off all the fat on my legs, but up to 15 km, everyday? That is obsessive behavior.

So instead, you can skip rope. Skip on an empty stomach. If you have eaten something, allow the food to digest for five hours, before you start jogging your body up and down skipping away.

Skipping also helps you get rid of that beer belly.

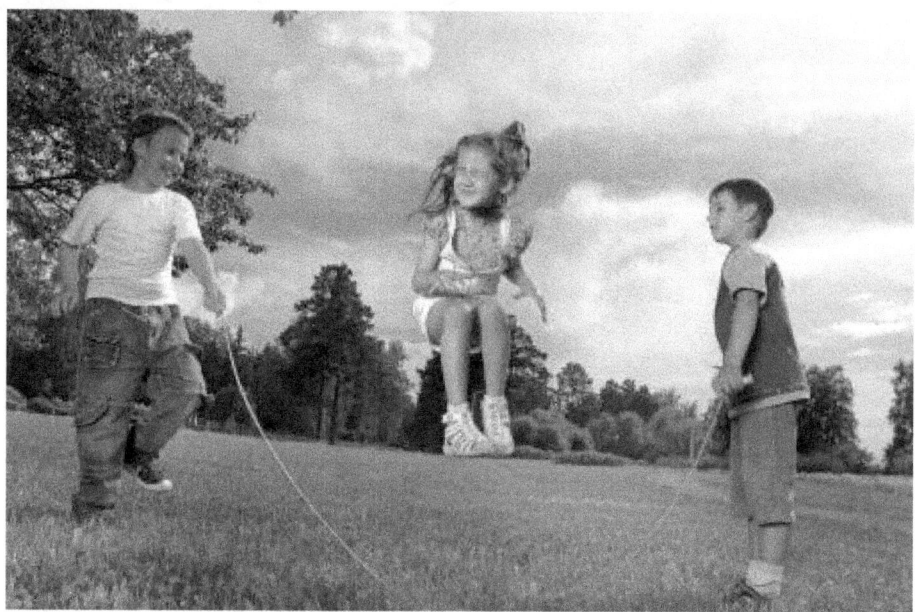

What fun!

Losing weight, all in one go is definitely not recommended. There are number of harmful weight loss fads going out on the Internet today, endorsed by anorexic superstars. And young children and teenagers are using them to lose weight. This is a very harmful practice, because this is the time when they need food in order to grow in a healthy manner. So if you have a teenager with an attitude of, I am going to go fat, I am not going to eat, you need to be very firm with him. Unless of course, he is already overweight due to bad eating habits inculcated in him during childhood.

That is when he will need to lose weight under the supervision of a doctor who is going to give him a good dietary plan to follow. Naturally you are going to supervise him and see that he follows this plan.

So it is going to take you a month to lose one kilogram of weight, in a healthy manner by brisk walking/jog trotting 3 mph every day.

Additional exercises are going to help you lose even more weight, as fatty tissue becomes muscular tissue.

Foods to Help You Lose Weight

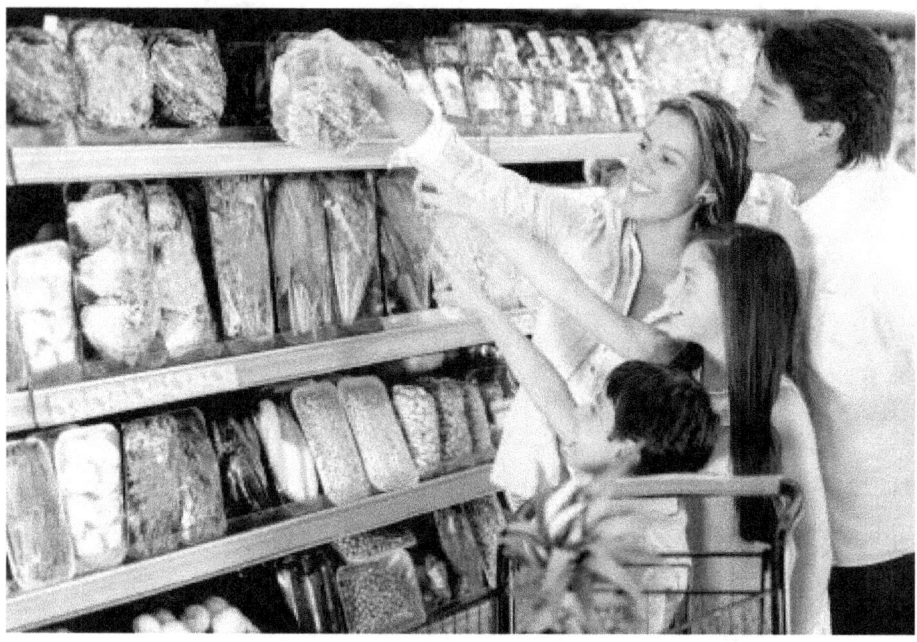

Fruit and vegetables have less of calories so start eating them more but do not eat bananas.

Do not add salt to your fruit salads, when you eat them. Also, stop eating sugary items, fried items and fatty items.

Try drinking mint tea. Tomatoes are excellent detox foods. A salad of raw tomatoes, with salt and onions every day is going to help reduce weight, especially when you eat it long-term. It is also going to detoxify your body.

Lemons – this is an ancient reducing remedy, which is still being followed in many parts of the world today. One lemon mixed with rock salt to taste in a glass full of hot water on an empty stomach, taken every day for two months is going to reduce your weight. Considerable weight loss can also be achieved with the juice of one lemon, one glass of hot water, and two spoonfuls of honey, for four months, especially in the hot season.

Spinach juice when taken with lemon is also a good weight-loss remedy.

Yogurt – yogurt with its probiotic bacteria is not only good for your system, but it is also helpful in helping you lose weight. That is the reason why so many dietitians recommending diet programs always insist of yogurt for breakfast or for lunch.

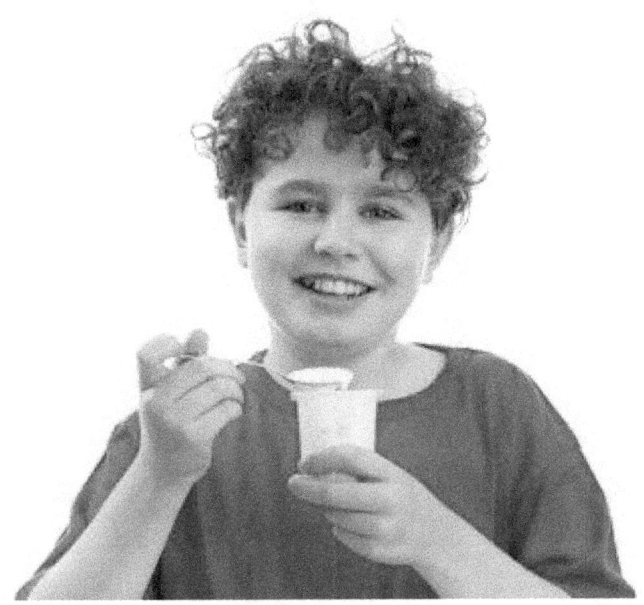

All right, let me tell you something which you may find very revolutionary. Potatoes in themselves do not help to increase weight. It is just that they are cooked in fat, and served heavy spiced. On the other hand, if you eat potatoes which have been boiled or have been roasted in hot sand, you are not going to find yourself getting fat. Try this out. Do not allow butter near these potatoes!

Try this lukewarm water remedy. Start drinking lukewarm water instead of ordinary water. Drink one glass of lukewarm water before eating anything. This stops you from feeling ravenously hungry. Two months of this remedy, and you are going to find yourself visibly losing weight.

You can also try this salt water remedy. Boil three glasses of water. Add a pinch full of salt to it. Drink a glass of this water in the morning on an empty stomach and then in the afternoon and then at night, before you go to sleep.

Also remember to drink one glass of hot water – as hot as you can bear, – as soon as you have finished your meal.

Permanent Weight Loss Remedy

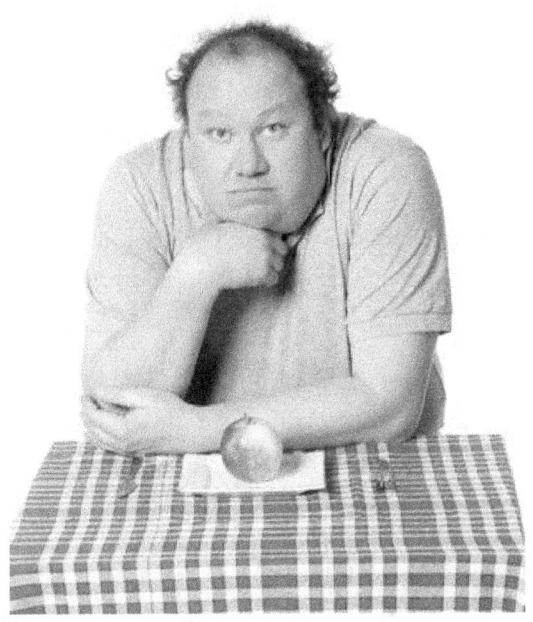

A weight loss regime does not mean depriving yourself of necessary nutrients.

This is a long-term treatment, which means that you are going to do it for up to four months, even though you can see the visible affects after 40 days.

For this you need to or three different types of seasonal fruit, lettuce leaves, radish, carrots, tomatoes, cabbage, ginger, green chilies, green coriander, lemon, mint leaves, black gram – which have been wet overnight – pepper and rock salt. Collect all these items according to availability and in needed portions you think appropriate.

Wash the lettuce leaves and the cabbage leaves and spread them all over your salad plate. Now cut the fruit and place them all over the leaves. You can slice the tomatoes and the radish, ginger and carrots can be made into julienne strips. Now add the black gram, which had been soaked overnight.

The third layer is going to be made of green coriander, mint leaves and green chilies. Sprinkle the lemon juice over them, and the rock salt and pepper to taste over this salad.

This is delicious and full of nutritional minerals. Finish this salad with your normal meal. You can also have it as an accompaniment to your afternoon tea. You can also use this dish instead of a dinner at night. Chew all the pieces well.

If you want to get rid of the weight around your stomach, waist, hips and thighs, have this salad instead of dinner. Also add tomato and spinach soup as an accompaniment.

It is going to take just 40 days for you to see a clearly visible reduction in your weight. You can reduce as much of weight as you want, with this method. This is a time-tested, and proven ancient remedy for weight loss.

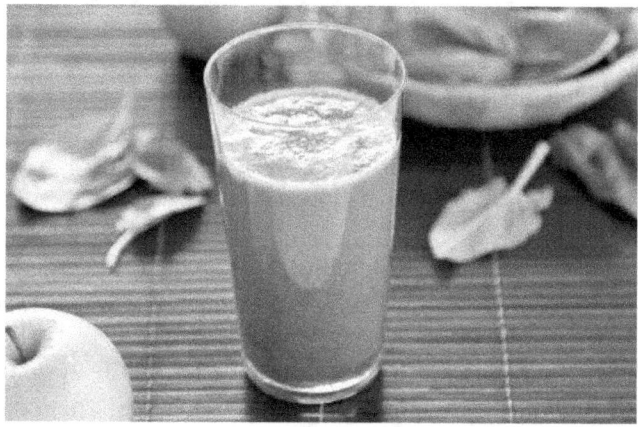

Spinach juice with lemon can help you to reduce weight.

Conclusion

This book is full of tips of healthy living, followed by the ancients to help keep you healthy and give you a long life.

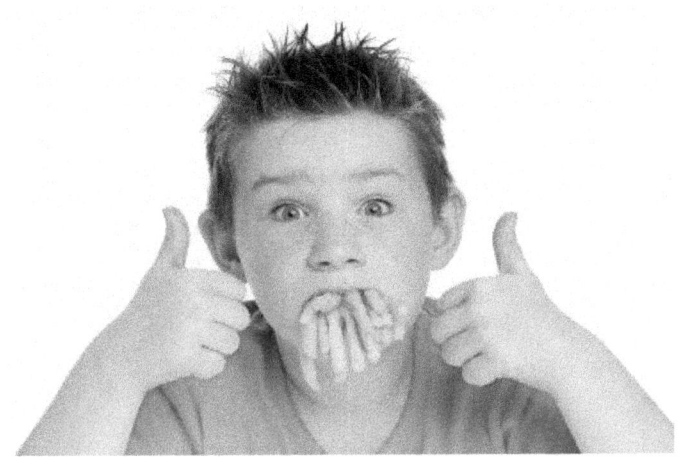

Talk about bad eating habits and food stuffing!

In the East, 40 days is a time period which means that at least you have been taking that particular treatment for more than a month. In many cases, a month is much more than sufficient to cure you. The 40 days meant that two risings and settings of the moon had taken place and the patient had been eating healing regular proper nutritive meal, during that time. 10 days were extra, just as an added booster and support to the 30 days of a month. The 40 day time period has had a religious and social significance, which most of us do not know, and which has been passed down to us down the ages.

I recommended four months because not only is it going to make you really slim and trim, but it is going to give you a glowing complexion. You are also going to find yourself eating less of junk and unhealthy food, and you are going to feel revitalized. Also, as it takes about one month for you to lose 1 kg of weight in a healthy manner – through the walking exercise of 3 mph for one hour, – four months mean about 4 kg – 8.8 pounds. Pretty good going, that.

The elders in the family even though they are in their 70s and 80s, now, have been eating this salad, ever since they were in their 40s. And they have never suffered from weight problems. They also have wonderful complexions and so much energy, that they are quite capable of putting the younger generation in the shade.

So, remember that these tips have come down to us from the ancients. Learn, Follow, Livelong And Prosper!

Author Bio

Dueep Jyot Singh is a Management and IT Professional who managed to gather Postgraduate qualifications in Management and English and Degrees in Science, French and Education while pursuing different enjoyable career options like being an hospital administrator, IT,SEO and HRD Database Manager/ trainer, movie , radio and TV scriptwriter, theatre artiste and public speaker, lecturer in French, Marketing and Advertising, ex-Editor of Hearts On Fire (now known as Solstice) Books Missouri USA, advice columnist and cartoonist, publisher and Aviation School trainer, ex-moderator on Medico.in, banker, student councilor ,travelogue writer … among other things!

One fine morning, she decided that she had enough of killing herself by Degrees and went back to her first love -- writing. It's more enjoyable! She already has 48 published academic and 14 fiction- in- different- genre books under her belt.

When she is not designing websites or making Graphic design illustrations for clients , she is browsing through old bookshops hunting for treasures, of which she has an enviable collection – including R.L. Stevenson, O.Henry, Dornford Yates, Maurice Walsh, De Maupassant, Victor Hugo, Sapper, C.N. Williamson, "Bartimeus" and the crown of her collection- Dickens "The Old Curiosity Shop," and so on… Just call her "Renaissance Woman") - collecting herbal remedies, acting like Universal Helping Hand/Agony Aunt, or escaping to her dear mountains for a bit of exploring, collecting herbs and plants and trekking.

Check out some of the other JD-Biz Publishing books

Gardening Series on Amazon

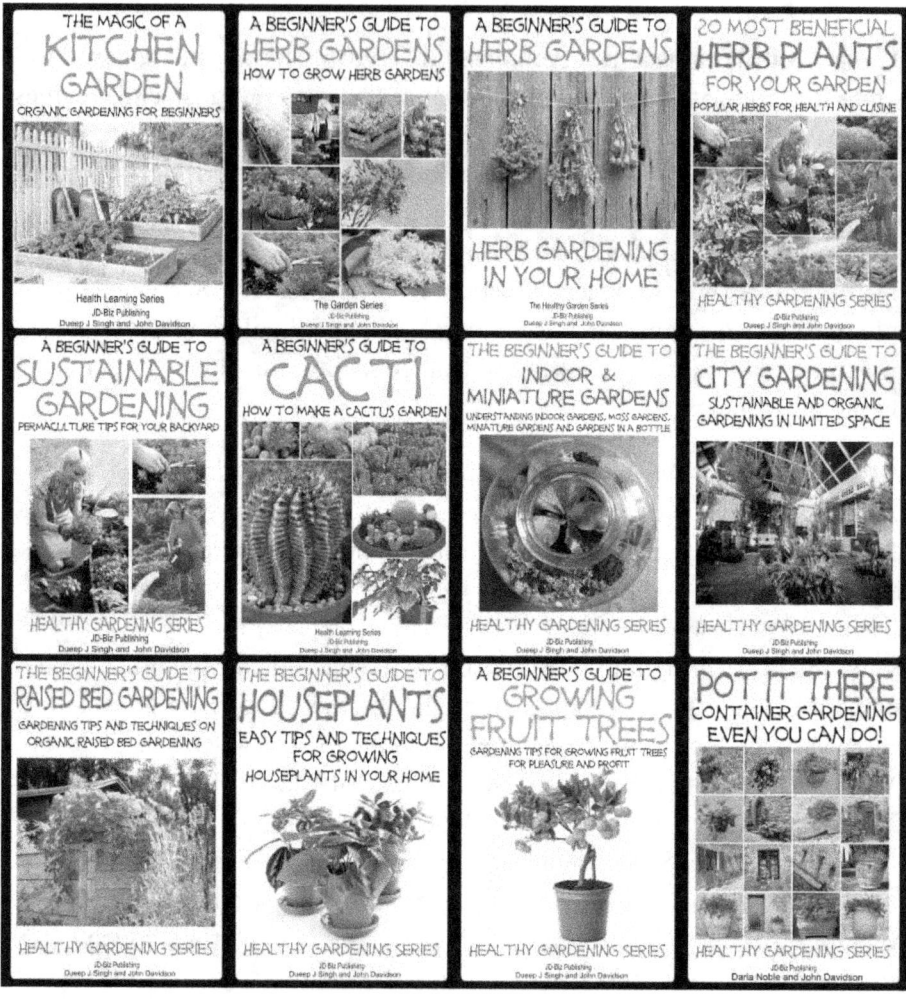

Health Learning Series

THE MAGIC OF GOOSEBERRIES FOR HEALTH AND BEAUTY	THE MAGIC OF YOGURT FOR COOKING AND BEAUTY	THE MAGIC OF LEMONS USING LEMONS FOR HEALTH AND BEAUTY	THE MAGIC OF CHILLIES FOR COOKING AND HEALING	THE MAGIC OF ONIONS ONIONS IN CUISINE TO CURE AND TO HEAL	THE MAGIC OF RADISHES TO CURE AND TO HEAL
THE MAGIC OF CARROTS TO CURE AND TO HEAL	THE HEALTH BENFITS OF OREGANO FOR COOKING AND HEALTH	The Magic of MARIGOLDS Marigolds for health And Beauty	THE HEALTH BENFITS OF CINNAMON FOR COOKING AND HEALTH	THE MAGIC OF COCONUTS FOR COOKING & HEALTH	THE MAGIC OF CLOVES FOR HEALING AND COOKING
THE MAGIC OF ASAFETIDA FOR COOKING AND HEALING	THE MAGIC OF NEEM MARGOSA TO HEAL	THE MAGIC OF SALT TO HEAL AND FOR BEAUTY	THE MAGIC OF POMEGRANATES FOR HEALTH AND BEAUTY	THE MAGIC OF DRY FRUIT AND SPICES REMEDIES AND RECIPES	THE HEALTH BENEFITS OF TURMERIC CURCUMIN FOR COOKING AND HEALTH
THE MAGIC OF ALOE VERA	THE MAGIC OF VEGETABLES ANCIENT HEALING REMEDIES AND TIPS	THE HEALTH BENEFITS OF ROSEMARY FOR COOKING AND HEALTH	THE MAGIC OF PEPPER & PEPPERCORNS FOR COOKING & HEALING	THE MAGIC OF MILK, BUTTER AND CHEESE FOR COOKING & HEALING	THE MAGIC OF CARDAMOMS FOR COOKING AND HEALTH
THE HEALTH BENEFITS OF BLACK CUMIN FOR COOKING AND HEALTH	THE MAGIC OF BASIL-TULSI TO HEAL NATURALLY	THE MAGIC OF SPICES FOR HEALTH AND CUISINE	THE MAGIC OF ROSES FOR COOKING AND BEAUTY	The Miraculous Healing Powers of GINGER	The Miracle of HONEY

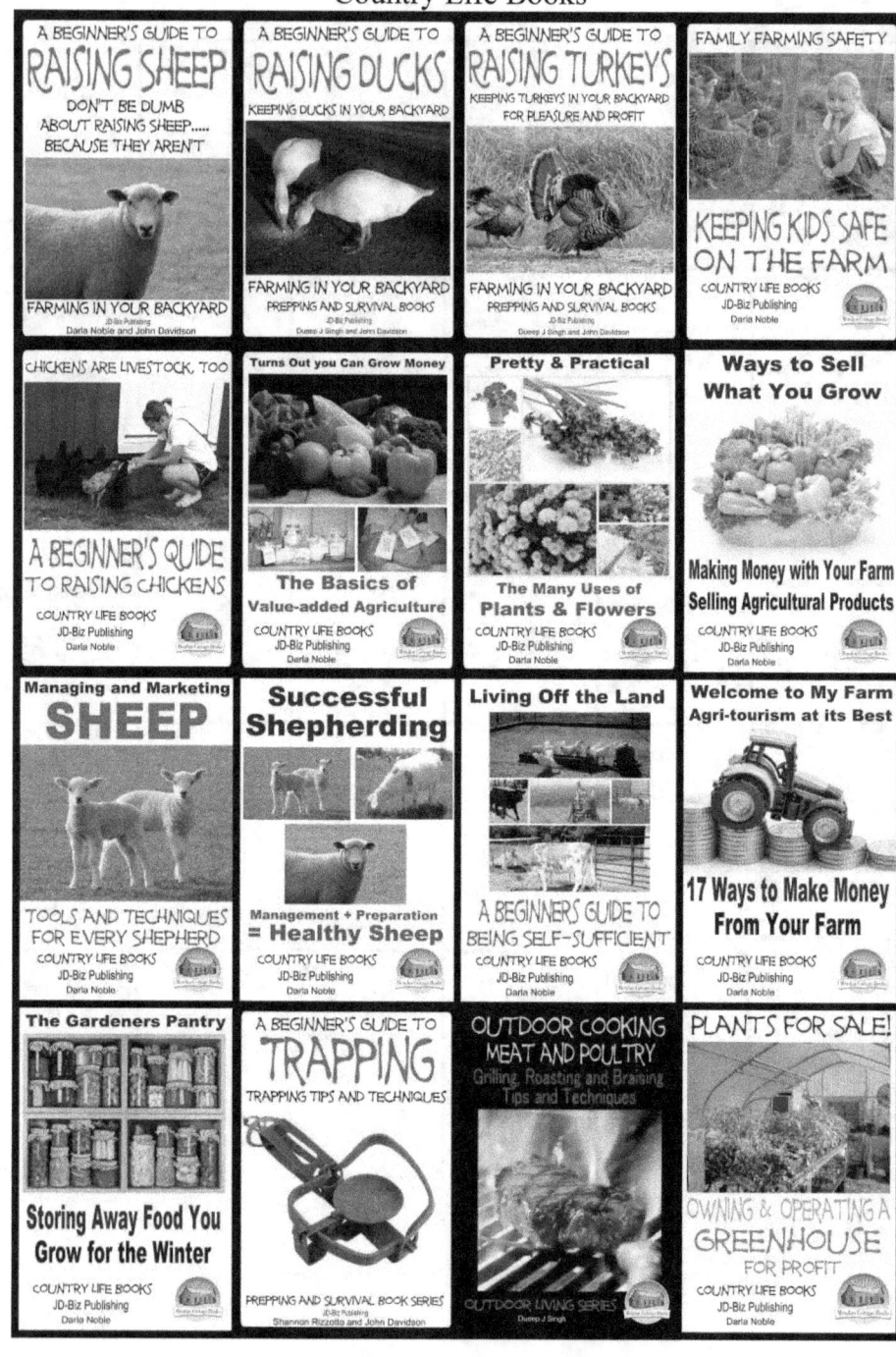

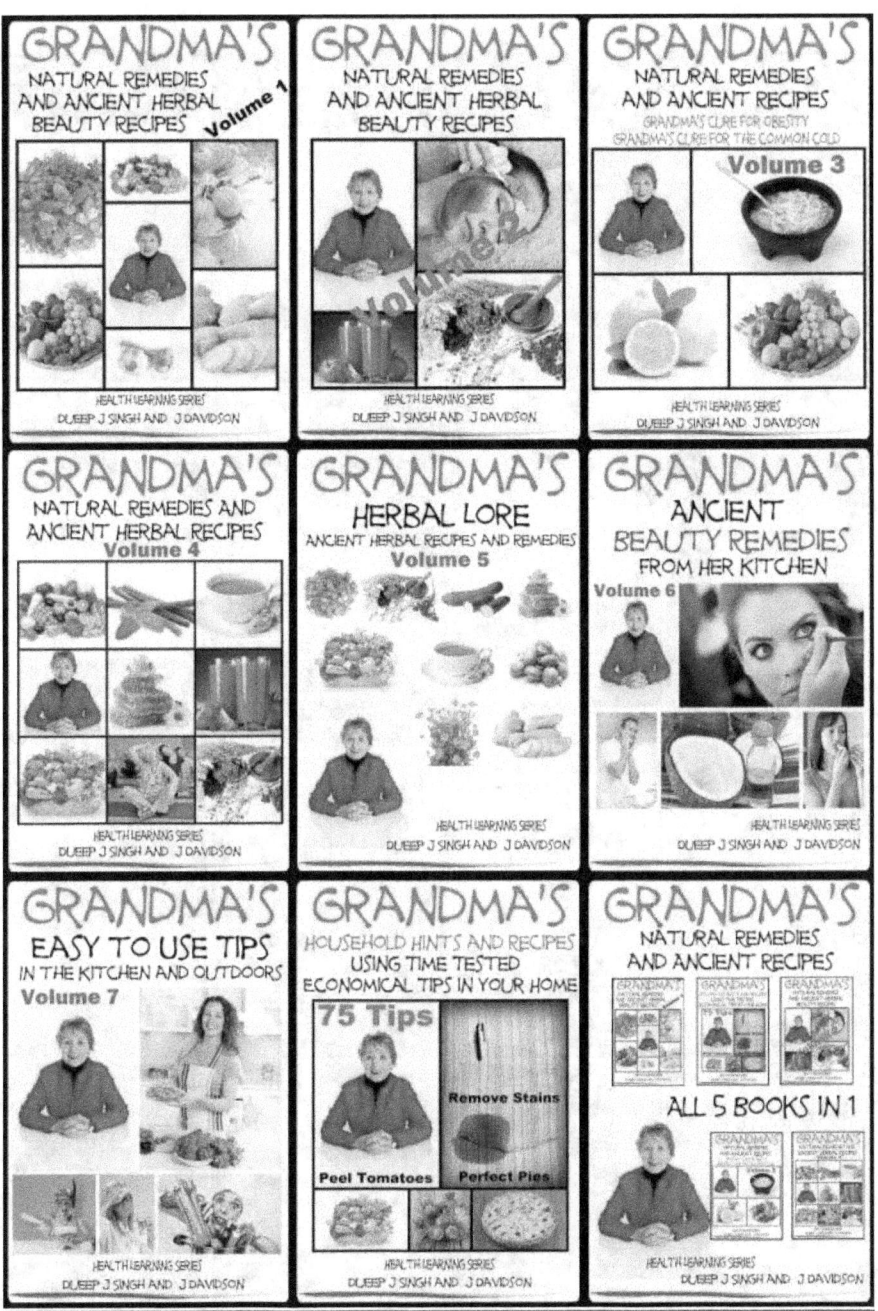

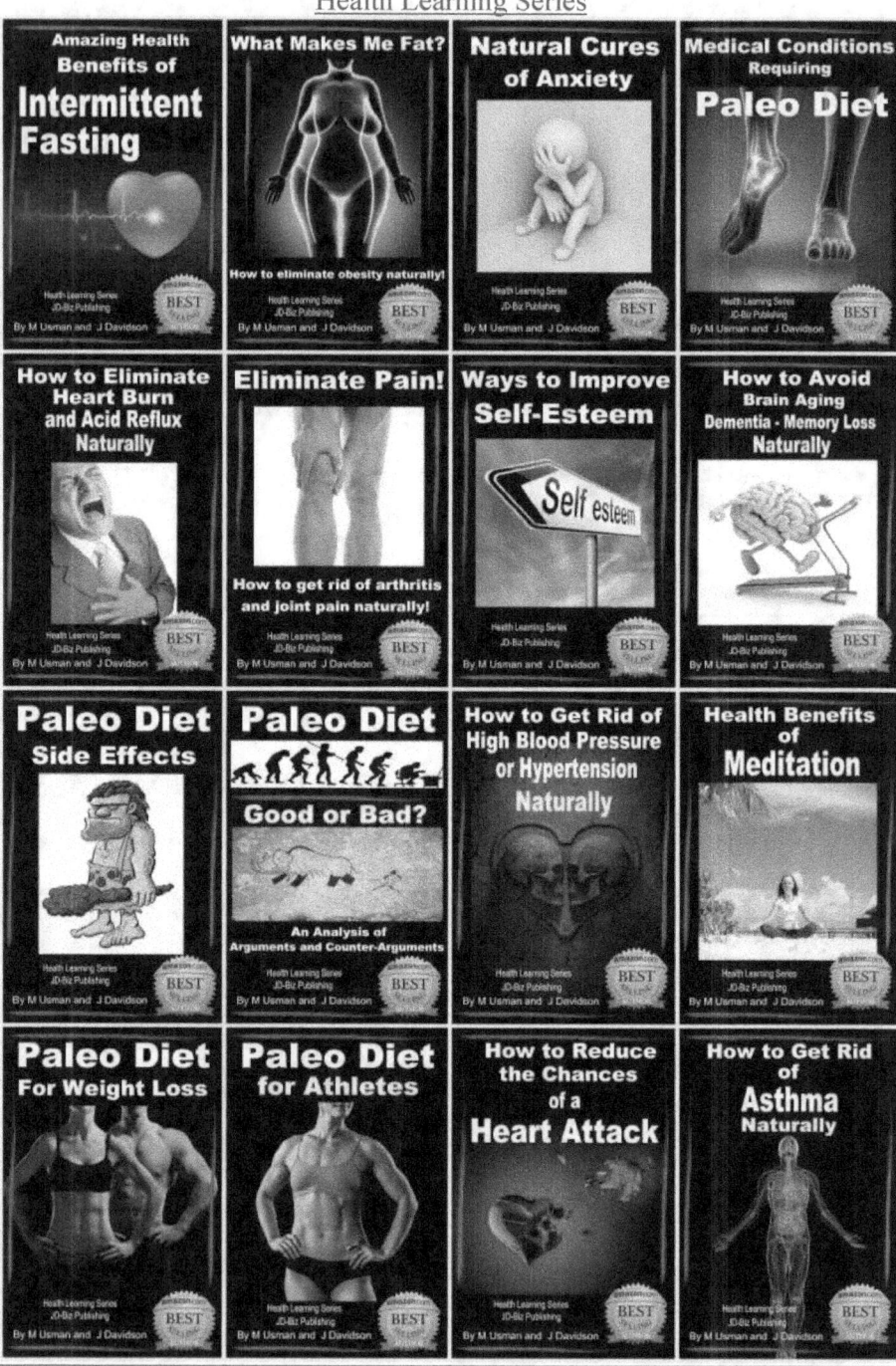

Amazing Animal Book Series

Learn To Draw Series

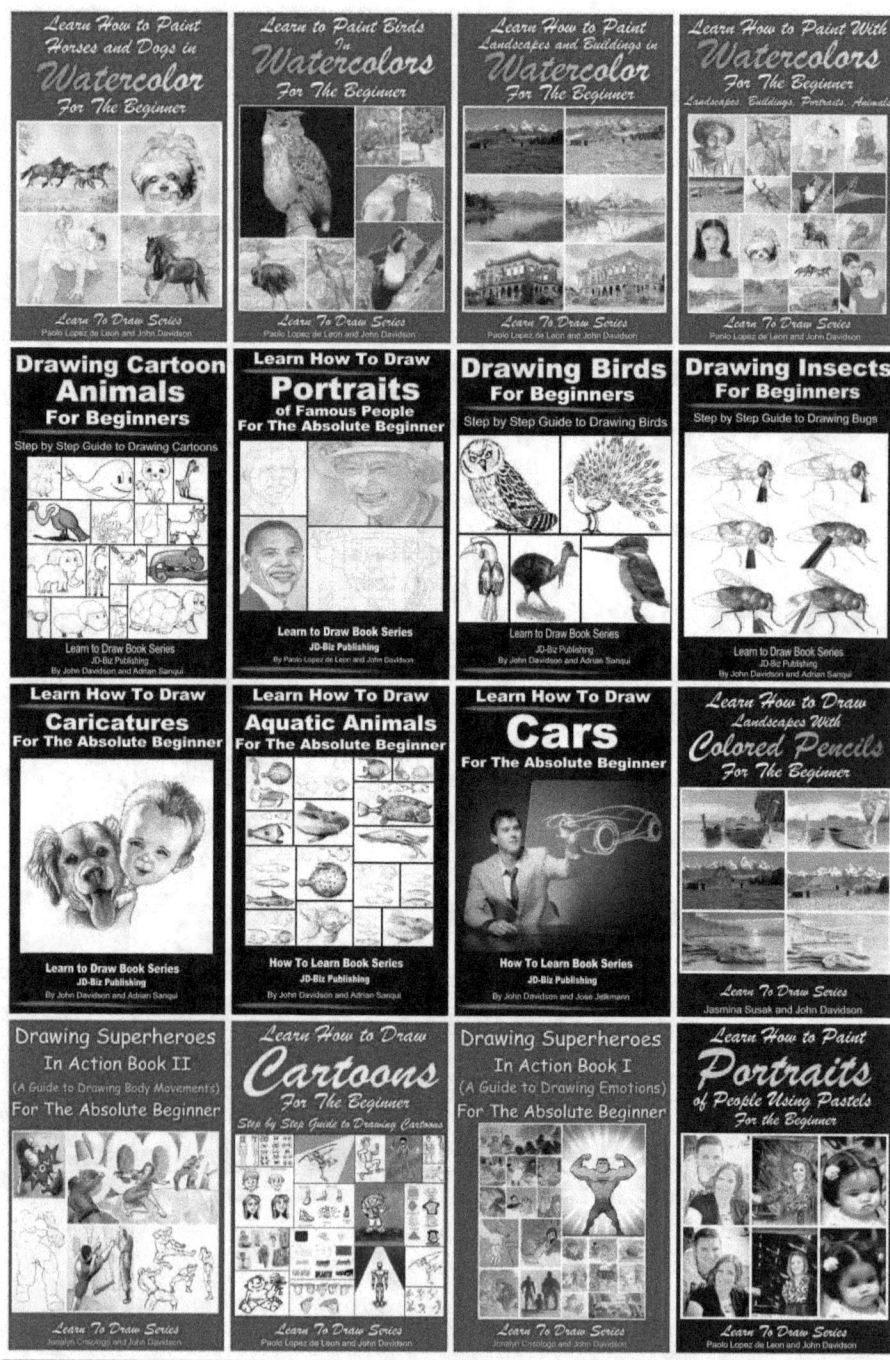

How to Build and Plan Books

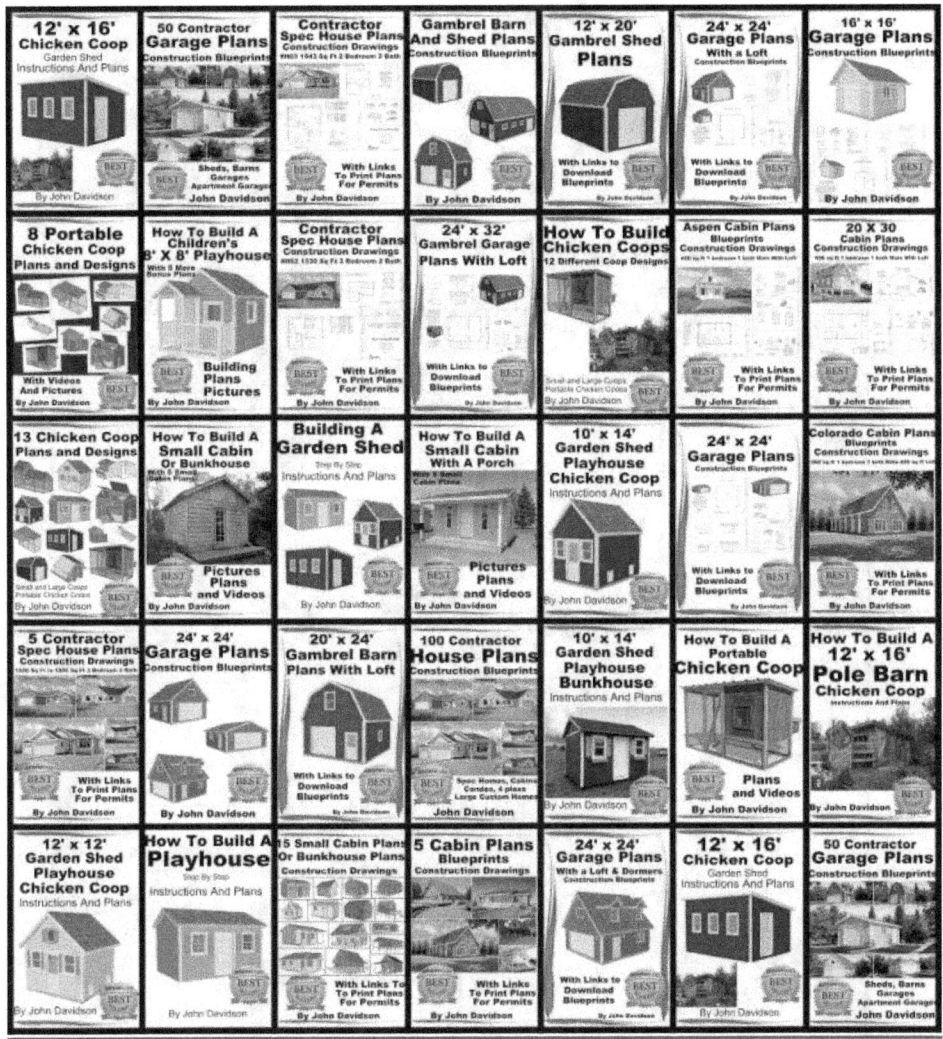

Entrepreneur Book Series

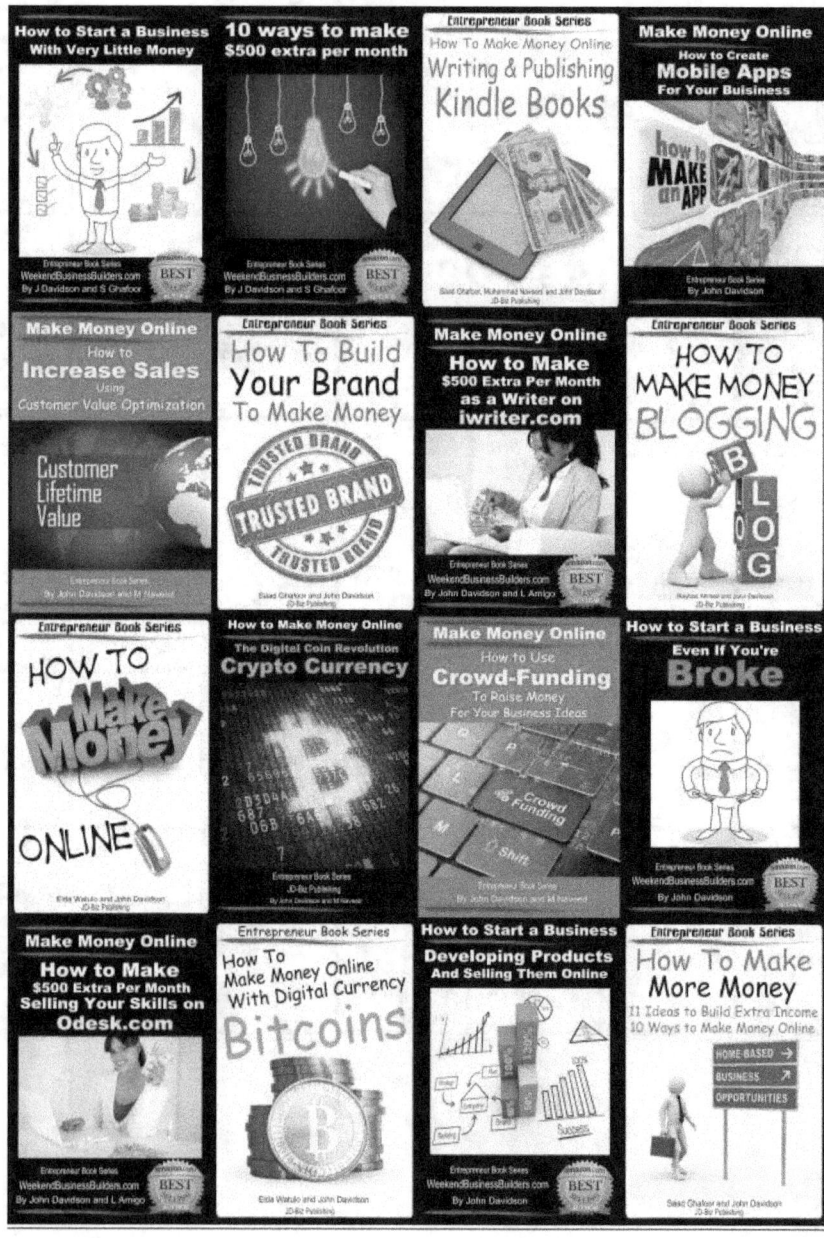

Our books are available at

1. Amazon.com

2. Barnes and Noble

3. Itunes

4. Kobo

5. Smashwords

6. Google Play Books

Publisher

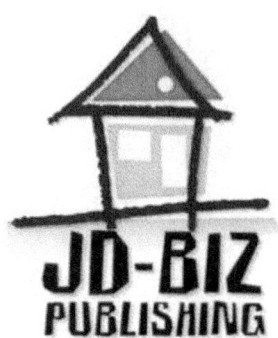

JD-Biz Corp

P O Box 374

Mendon, Utah 84325

http://www.jd-biz.com/

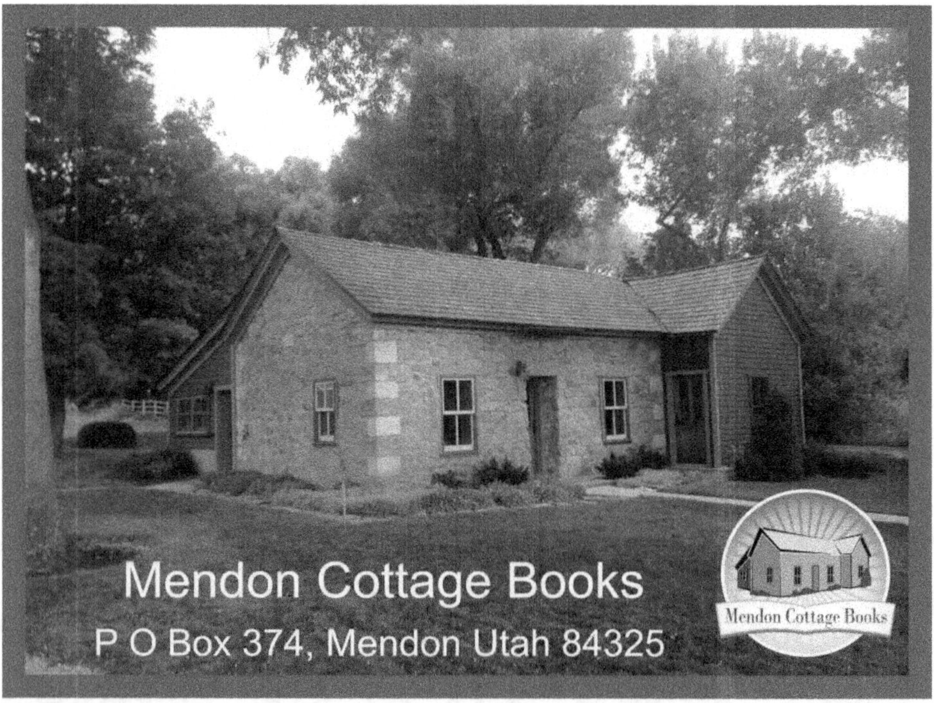

Mendon Cottage Books

P O Box 374, Mendon Utah 84325

Mendon Cottage Books

www.ingramcontent.com/pod-product-compliance
Lightning Source LLC
Chambersburg PA
CBHW070625290526
45790CB00002B/991